Seven Weeks
to Sobriety

Seven Weeks to Sobriety

The Proven Program to Fight Alcoholism through Nutrition

(Formerly titled: *Alcoholism—The Biochemical Connection:
A Breakthrough Seven-Week Self-Treatment Program*)

Joan Mathews Larson, Ph.D.

Fawcett Columbine
New York

A Fawcett Columbine Book
Published by Ballantine Books

Library of Congress Catalog Card Number: 93-72173

ISBN: 0-449-90896-8

Cover design by Judy Herbstman

Manufactured in the United States of America

First Ballantine Books Edition: January 1994

10 9 8

To my husband, Ralph,
who empowered my work with
his love and financial support.

Foreword

The basic assumptions of most of the people who treat alcoholism have changed relatively little in the nearly 40 years I have practiced medicine. The assumption then, as now, is that if alcoholics would only get their act together, they would recover from their affliction.

Now, I don't want to sound like a complete pessimist, for there have been many significant medical advances. In my home state, where the Minnesota Model of alcoholism care was developed and fostered, the professionals at the Johnson Institute, Hazelden Foundation, St. Mary's Hospital, and other facilities have taken important steps.

These efforts to improve care of this disease have made people more understanding about the plight of alcoholics. Employers' attitudes have changed, and insurance now often covers the treatment of alcoholism. Churches and faith communities now open their doors for meetings of support groups like Alcoholics Anonymous or other twelve-step programs, such as those begun by Dr. Vern Bittner of the Institute for Christian Living in Minneapolis, a program based on the AA model of reflection and understanding.

Colleges and universities offer classes and courses concerning substance abuse and addiction. And families and individuals can now talk more openly about alcoholism and can rely on community resources that provide services all the way from Al-Anon to detox units.

The federal government now funds basic research at the National Institute on Alcohol Abuse and Alcoholism. Private groups have come together to form the National Council on Alcoholism.

The medical community now recognizes the need for specialists in this area. They have formed the American Society of Addiction Medicine (ASAM), which is based in Washington, D.C. ASAM conducts national conferences and workshops, publishes newsletters, educational material, and the *Journal of Addictive Diseases,* and sponsors a wide range of other activities.

Despite all these developments, success in curing alcoholism remains elusive. Nearly 80 percent of alcoholics receiving treatment relapse within one or two years. Didn't these people try hard enough? Didn't their spouses or families do the right things? Did their bosses expect too much and push them too hard?

Such questions always aroused my curiosity. Perhaps this is what made me say yes when Joan Mathews Larson, Ph.D., the founder of Health Recovery Center (HRC) in Minneapolis and author of this book, called me in 1985 and asked me to be medical consultant for HRC. I served in this capacity for over six years.

When I accepted the position, I was a typically uninformed physician. I had learned the usual information given to us in medical school and printed in our scientific journals. I accepted the standard doctrine that alcoholism was primarily—if not exclusively—a psychological dysfunction.

I had visited alcoholism treatment centers and alcoholism wards at the local and state hospitals. I knew that the primary treatment consisted of having the patient abstain from alcohol and participate in group and one-on-one counseling. The insiders, both patients and professionals, accepted this head talk as usual and customary fare.

The methods and degree of confrontation used varied from place to place and counselor to counselor. Many seemed to go in for the same sort of shock treatment given out by big, tough marine sergeants in boot camp. Others were less aggressive. I saw tears being shed and personalities hung out to dry in front of everyone. I heard the common pleas and claims:

"My wife made me drink."

"My kids make me angry."

"My husband makes me so mad I need a drink."

"My boss treats me so bad I need a couple of cocktails after work to calm down."

After the finger pointing and accusations wore down and the patients grew a little more sophisticated and outspoken, I began to hear these questions:

"Does this demeaning type of encounter really help?"

"Why do they insist on all this digging through the manure?"

"Why does a minor tiff with my spouse change me?"

"Is my biochemistry or metabolic makeup different?"

"Why am I so *vulnerable?*"

As I began to examine more and more patients in my first two years at HRC, I began to see certain patterns. The majority of patients suffered from one (or more) of five disorders:

1. Nutritional deficits of such substances as B-complex vitamins, basic amino acids, and key minerals such as zinc, magnesium, and calcium

2. Food allergies to everyday table items such as corn, wheat, and dairy products

3. Thyroid disorders, most often what we call subclinical hypothyroidism, or "sluggish thyroid"

4. Hypoglycemia (low blood sugar) that caused a wide range of poorly understood symptoms (anxiety, fatigue, depression, panic attacks)

5. Candida-related complex (CRC), a mysterious but common disorder resulting from an overgrowth of the yeast *Candida albicans* (this condition is often triggered by excessive use of broad-spectrum antibiotics for such conditions as sinusitis,

bronchitis, and upper-respiratory infections related to heavy smoking, all common problems for alcoholics)

I began to speculate that one or more of these other factors might be the missing pieces of the puzzle. That brought me back to the premise that alcoholism is not *primarily* a psychological disorder. But how does it all fit together?

There is no doubt that alcoholics do experience such symptoms as moodiness, irritability, insomnia, depression, anxiety, and fatigue. No doubt these have psychological ramifications, but are they the *causes* of alcoholism or merely the *symptoms* of other medical problems?

Dr. Larson had done extensive research on the nutritional status of her patients and associated allergies and food sensitivities, and treatment for these disorders had helped her patients make dramatic improvements. However, there were still other variables to be considered. Complex metabolic roller coasters were still at work.

It became clear to me and other members of the HRC staff that just as *no amount of psychological counseling* could talk a diabetic out of his or her metabolic disorder, psychological *counseling* of alcoholics was not enough. Successful treatment required proper medical intervention, dietary counseling, meal planning, and similar efforts. Psychological counseling and support can help both the alcoholic and the diabetic, but head talk alone can't provide a cure.

At HRC, we felt that the reason for the poor success rate (20 percent) in traditional alcoholism treatment programs (versus 75 percent at HRC) was due to the failure to treat the *other* problems that mask themselves as "psychological."

Unfortunately, in over 90 percent of our nation's treatment programs, the *psychological model persists*. The mind-set of the traditional alcoholic/chemical dependency professional is hard to change. An example of this reluctance to change was the one I experienced with a physician who is prominent in our local alcoholism treatment community.

I asked Dr. X to cover for me at HRC while I was out of town on a lecture trip. He was most cordial and agreed to help the first time. However, when I requested his services for a second time, he wrote me, "No, I can't do it. Your patients and staff seem to be so negative about the care provided in other treatment programs and so gung ho about HRC that I was uncomfortable being there!"

Dr. X's dilemma about this different view of alcoholism reminds me of an article that I read in the *Journal of the American Medical Association* (J. S. and J. M. Goodwin: "The Tomato Effect: Rejection of Highly Effective Therapies"). The authors, a husband-and-wife team from the University of New Mexico School of Medicine, explained that the "Tomato Effect," a phenomenon that originally occurred in a rural community in New Jersey over a common fruit now known to be a safe and useful crop, also occurs in the medical community. Highly efficacious treatment for a certain problem is rejected or ignored because it doesn't "make sense" in the light of accepted theories of diseases and medical practice. They reported, "The tomato was ignored because it was described as 'clearly poisonous.' " It belonged to the nightshade *(solanaceae)* family, of whose members, belladonna and mandrake, for example, have leaves and fruit that are known to cause death if ingested in sufficient quantity. Because of that, during the eighteenth century tomatoes were not eaten or even cultivated in North America.

It was not until 1820 that Robert Gibbon Johnson, a farmer from Salem, New Jersey, demonstrated to other farmers and townspeople, by eating tomatoes on the front steps of the county courthouse each week, that the fruit was not poisonous. "Only then did the people of America grudgingly, we suspect, begin to consume tomatoes." The Goodwins then concluded, "Commercial cultivation of tomatoes was rare until the twentieth century, although in the past eight decades, the tomato has grown to become our *largest cash crop.*"

We hope that this book will increase awareness that treatment for alcoholism has to be changed and broadened. The methods presented here are safe and effective. The breakthrough is the recognition that alcoholism has many biochemical connections and that head talk alone will not work for most patients.

The hundreds of thousands of people with the black cloud of alcoholism hanging over their heads should throw away the guilt and the anxiety and the misconceptions they have about their alcoholism or that of their loved ones. When they understand that alcoholism, like diabetes, is a physiological disorder, there is more acceptance, less confusion, and far less guilt. Most alcoholics are glad to learn that they were born with certain biochemical vulnerabilities and that minimizing or treating these conditions is a safer bet than trying to cure the mysterious psychological weaknesses that have for decades been assumed to be the cause of alcoholism.

Most people accept the fact that our genes affect our looks and health. Some people have bad feet. Some inherit weak eyes, funny noses, or big ears. Others have bad allergies that flare up at certain times of the year or are present, unfortunately, nearly all the time.

Similarly, in certain families there are more alcoholics than would be expected. Certain inheritable traits or biotypes can cause the cases of alcoholism that are not strictly psychological in origin.

I once questioned an HRC patient about alcoholism in his family. He said, "Mom was fine, but of my seven brothers and sisters, all but one are alcoholics. My dad was a drunk and died behind a dumpster near skid row. Boy, did I pick the wrong family."

This book is a terrific resource not only for such patients, but for their families and counselors as well. The insights offered are truly breakthroughs. The methods described are on the cutting edge of knowledge about alcoholism, its causes and cases. It will provide much in the way of individual help and could also greatly reduce the cost and misery that alcoholism causes for our citizens, cities, states, and for our nation as a whole.

It is my hope—and Dr. Larson's—that this book will help diminish the skepticism that has delayed wider acceptance of the principles practiced at HRC and described in the following pages.

Our program's twelve years of success in Minnesota can now be shared with you. It is my hope and prayer that this book will lead to a new Minnesota Model for the treatment and cure of alcoholism. It's about time!

KEITH W. SEHNERT, M.D.

Acknowledgments

My grateful thanks to the many biochemists, physicians, and researchers whose combined works have provided the basis for this treatment model.

A special thank-you to:

Dr. Keith Sehnert, Health Recovery Center's medical director, who encouraged the writing of this book and spent many hours assisting with the medical directions contained herein;

Dr. Tom Wittkopp, HRC's supervising psychiatrist for nine years, who lent his knowledge and support through the rough times;

Jean Schoeberl, program director since HRC's inception, whose contributions both to this treatment model and to my emotional health are priceless;

Robert Parker, coauthor of HRC's research study, who gave us many years of his genius before his untimely death;

Molly Mathews, whose commitment to this work is as great as my own;

And all of my colleagues at HRC, who have worked tirelessly to bring about this treatment breakthrough.

Contents

Introduction

Alcoholism is not a character defect. It is not the sign of a weak will. It is not a bad habit that needs to be broken. It is a devastating physical disease that damages both mind and body. But recovery is possible. This book offers you a proven, seven-week treatment program that will put an end to your addiction to alcohol and restore your physical and emotional health. I have spent the past ten years testing and fine-tuning this approach with hundreds of alcoholics. The results speak for themselves: more than 75 percent of those treated at Health Recovery Center have broken their addiction to alcohol, maintained their sobriety, and regained their health. With traditional treatment methods, only 15 to 25 percent recover.

Alcoholism—The Biochemical Connection will help you stop drinking and detoxify your body with minimal discomfort. It will also help you put a permanent end to your craving for alcohol, rebuild your physical and emotional health, and abolish the depression that so often accompanies alcoholism.

If all this sounds too good to be true, let me assure you that this book is based on solid research by some of the world's most distinguished scientists. My staff and I developed the program at Health Recovery Center, an outpatient treatment facility in Minneapolis. We have treated more than one thousand clients from all over the United States, and our unprecedented success has generated an enormous amount of interest from treatment professionals around the world. Many are beginning to adopt our methods, but knowing how desperate alcoholics are for treatment that works, I decided to write this book in order to make the program immediately available to a wide audience.

Alcoholism—The Biochemical Connection gives you the following promises:

- You will be able to determine if you have addictive chemistry and are at risk for alcoholism
- You will discover how to break your addiction with minimal discomfort
- You will get the tools you need to turn off alcohol cravings once and for all
- You'll discover the joy of abolishing depression and other unstable moods
- You'll use state-of-the-art methods to rebuild a high level of physical and emotional health for yourself

And your timetable for applying these proven tools is seven short weeks.

Your chances of success are excellent if you simply follow the book's instructions. You'll share the same protocol for wellness, the same how-to charts and tests, the same detoxification methods and repair formulas that have healed so many before you.

It is exhilarating to be in charge of your life again. If you follow the program as presented in this book, in seven weeks you'll be able to put alcoholism behind you, pick up the pieces of your life, and move forward, with newfound vigor and optimism, to a bright and healthy future.

Seven Weeks
to Sobriety

One

Loss of a Son, Birth of a Concept

I know you want to recover from alcoholism. I have met few alcoholics who were not desperate to stop drinking. Many try and most fail. If you are one of them, I expect you to be somewhat skeptical of the very idea of a treatment breakthrough that can lead to permanent recovery. You may not believe that any treatment can banish the overpowering craving for alcohol that has defeated all your past efforts. You may not even want to believe it.

But permanent recovery is possible. The breakthrough I describe in this book can liberate you from alcoholism, free you from cravings, restore your health, and help you overcome depression or other emotional problems underlying your drinking. I know those are bold promises, and I would not make them if I wasn't very sure that this program can help you. For the past ten years I have tested, retested, and fine-tuned this approach. It works. It has worked for more than one thousand alcoholics. And it will work for you.

The program itself is based on solid scientific research that challenges all the old assumptions about the very nature of alcoholism. This research conclusively demonstrates that alcoholism is a physical disease, rooted in the genes and activated by the effect of alcohol on the biochemistry of the brain and body. An enormous number of well-controlled scientific studies by distinguished researchers the world over has shown that alcohol undermines physical health and mental stability by destroying the vital nutrients responsible for their maintenance. Additional studies have shown that alcoholism can be conquered by undoing this damage.

And that, in a nutshell, is the concept that underlies this plan. In seven short weeks I will help you fix what alcohol has broken. Unlike other treatment programs, this plan is based on physical repair. As you read the pages ahead, you will learn a lot about the natural chemistry that governs your body and your brain. I'm certain that you will be impressed by the weight of scientific evidence and will quickly come to appreciate the importance of repairing the damage alcohol can inflict on your delicate internal chemistry.

Once you begin the program you'll notice a difference in the way you feel almost immediately. You'll be delighted at how easy it is to stop drinking with the aid of the nutrient-packed detoxification formula that blocks cravings for alcohol. Then, I'll show you how to individualize a repair program to restore your physical and emotional health.

I have been using this program to treat alcoholics since 1981, when I founded Health Recovery Center to test my theory that physical rehabilitation was the missing link in the treatment of alcoholism. Since then, I have treated more than one thousand alcoholics and drug addicts. More than three-quarters remain successfully rehabilitated and abstinent. You may not realize it, but a 75 percent recovery rate is unheard of in this field. Elsewhere, success rates are a dismal 25 percent. Our success has attracted attention from all over the world. Almost daily I receive calls from treatment directors and counselors anxious to learn about our methods. I can't take full credit for this breakthrough, which is based on the work of many respected researchers. I simply took their findings and put them into practice.

I didn't set out to find a new way to treat alcoholism; the events of my life led me to it. Twenty years ago, my husband had a heart attack and died at age forty. Suddenly, I was a single parent with nothing more practical than a degree in art with which to support my three children. Rob, my middle child, was thirteen at the time. He seemed most affected by the devastating change in our lives. "We just don't feel like a family anymore," he told me again and again.

Rob had always been an active boy with a wide range of interests. Before his father's death, his grades were excellent, he won leading roles in school plays, and played halfback for Tait's Tigers, a neighborhood football team. He was also notably softhearted and fair-minded. He championed the civil rights of the few minority students in his nearly all-white suburban elementary school and volunteered to help youngsters in the lower grades with their reading.

After the shock of my husband's death wore off, Rob's mood swings became more noticeable. So did his love for junk food and colas. Of course, we didn't use the term "junk food" back in 1972. Americans were still relatively naïve about nutrition, and the slogan "you are what you eat" conjured up images of the radical fringes of the fruit and nut bunch in California.

I had more on my mind at the time than the amount of cola my kids were drinking. I realized that I would have to go back to school for another, more useful degree in order to support my family. Rob was fifteen when I returned to college to study psychology. Following my classroom work I served two counseling internships in alcohol- and drug-dependency treatment programs. By then, Rob was a high school student developing a liking for "keggers," outdoor beer parties popular among teenagers in our area. His frequent partying coincided with my growing interest in chemical dependency. Ironically, as he moved farther and farther down the path of alcohol abuse, he was teaching me my life's work.

During my internships, I read some fascinating research by the endocrinologist John Tintera, M.D., a charter member of the New York State Commission on Alcoholism. Tintera's work focused on the relationship between low blood sugar (hypoglycemia) and alcohol abuse. The symptoms he described—shakiness, mood swings, irritability, emotional instability, sudden fatigue, mental confusion—sounded a lot like what Rob had been experiencing. Tintera explained that blood sugar, or glucose, is the brain's only fuel; when brain glucose levels drop, these uncomfortable symptoms develop. In a hypoglycemic person, a sudden infusion of glucose (in the form of sugars contained in candy bars, high-sugar colas, or alcoholic drinks) taken to relieve these symptoms triggers an abnormally large response of insulin, which counteracts the effects of glucose and creates a mild insulin shock. Tintera was the first to suggest that habitual alcohol consumption can actually create hypoglycemia by continually triggering insulin reactions.

I wondered whether Rob was in the grips of this feast-or-famine problem. Eventually, I decided to stop guessing and took him for a six-hour glucose tolerance test. The results showed that Rob was seriously hypoglycemic. At the time, much of his life revolved around ingesting sugars, particularly alcohol, a sugar that reaches the brain quite rapidly. Drinking gave him energy and made him feel great, and he never followed the doctor's advice to cut down on alcohol, or on colas and sweets.

I knew Rob needed help. His mood swings were becoming more marked and his grades were declining. I enrolled him in a highly recommended hospital inpatient alcohol treatment program for adolescents. I felt enormous relief when he was admitted. I had turned my worries over to the experts. Surely they could help.

The program focused on identifying the underlying psychological reasons for Rob's drinking. The counselors fixed on his relationship with his father and assumed that Rob's drinking problems stemmed from feelings of guilt—all the things he had or hadn't said to his father in the months before my husband's death. In retrospect, I can see that Rob eventually came to believe that he felt guilty and that his guilt led him to drink.

Hospital rules forbade Rob to come home, so I could see him only when I took part in group therapy. During these sessions, the counselors reproached me for telling Rob that I loved him whether or not he drank. The program's approach was more conditional: "If you do this (stop drinking), then I will do this (love you)." That didn't work for me or for Rob. He was very lonely, and I wasn't surprised when, a week before Christmas, the hospital notified me that Rob and a friend had left.

After a day-long drinking spree, Rob tried to sneak into the house through his bedroom window. When I found him and confronted him, he refused to return to the hospital. His counselors advised me to have him escorted back by the police. I was still convinced that the program would help and that I had no choice but to do as they suggested. But I began to have second thoughts when two policemen wrestled my son into submission and dragged him out of the house. Rob seemed strangely dazed. I now realize he was in insulin shock from drinking so much and not eating all day.

Instead of taking him back to the hospital, the police took Rob to the juvenile detention center, where he spent the weekend. He returned to the hospital just before Christmas.

I will never forget that Christmas Day. My other two children, Mark, then eighteen, and Molly, twelve, packed up Rob's presents, and we drove to the hospital. Throughout the day we heard the sobbing of another youngster locked in the "quiet room." She cried the whole afternoon. That Christmas was one of the saddest, most punishing days of my life.

Rob was considered a difficult case. His counselors were frustrated by his failure to break down and pour out his anger and shame. Finally, Rob understood what he had to do to gain his release. He learned to get in touch with his feelings so intensely that he didn't waste time with underlying reasons but became angry or depressed over every event in his life.

With this "progress," he earned his release. However, his counselors advised against his coming home. Instead, they recommended that he spend the next six months in a halfway house. I had misgivings. As a boy, Rob had been miserable with homesickness during the two weeks he spent at summer camp, but I felt I had no other choice than to trust the experts and the state-of-the-art treatment they offered.

I will never forget one family-therapy session at the halfway house. Rob and I were sitting with other parents and kids in a circle on the floor, getting in touch with our feelings. Rob became hysterical and began to weep over a minor issue. His mood swing was inexplicable. I began to wonder whether we were on the right track. He seemed almost worse than before treatment began.

Rob remained at the halfway house until the end of August. Then he came home and began his senior year in high school. Life seemed to be returning to normal. He was happy to be home at last and eager to return to school activities. On the day he died, two weeks after the beginning of the school year, he went to see his guidance counselor to make sure he would have enough credits to graduate. He was elated to learn that he did.

That night Rob and his friend Bruce sat up talking until early morning. Then he came into my room and woke me. "I love you," he said. "I'm sorry for the trouble I've been, but it will be okay from now on." After he left, I dozed off, relieved at how much better he seemed. But before breakfast, Mark heard the car motor running in the garage. He found Robby lying under the exhaust pipe. We rushed him to the hospital, but he was declared dead on arrival.

Rob's death was a personal tragedy, but it was not the isolated event I believed it to be. Recent research shows that nearly 25 percent of deaths among those treated for chemical dependency are the result of suicide. The psychiatrists who had treated Rob during the eight months that he was away from home never mentioned depression. Yet I had seen him depressed many times within a single day as his moods swung from high to low. Just hours before his death he had been thrilled at the news that he would graduate from high school on time. He had then quickly become depressed enough to take his life. How much more clear could the evidence of unstable brain chemistry be?

If I had known then what I know now about the chemical relationship between heavy alcohol use and depression, I might have been able to save my son.

In the fifteen years since Rob's death, I have been searching for a more effective and humane approach to treating alcoholism. I tried to read everything available on the subject and was stunned to learn that only 15 to 25 percent of alcoholics treated actually recover and that many, like Rob, commit suicide. As I read, I began to wonder why alcoholism, which is now considered a physical disease, is treated only psychologically.

I wanted to know more about the role Rob's hypoglycemia played in his alcohol dependency. I found an impressive amount of research on the effect of alcohol on a number of crucial brain chemicals and learned that alcohol-induced depletion of these vital substances can distort perception and cause anxiety, confusion, and depression, the very symptoms psychologically based treatment programs assume cause alcoholics to drink. Eventually I came to the conclusion that traditional approaches to the treatment of alcoholism were missing the point. Couldn't much of the hopelessness and depression, the violent mood swings and other psychological symptoms be the *effects* of heavy alcohol use rather than its cause?

In 1978 two other therapists and I received funding from the National Institute on Alcohol Abuse and Alcoholism to establish a chemical-dependency program at the Chrysalis Center for Women in Minneapolis. There we routinely ran glucose tolerance tests on all our clients and were amazed to find that more than three-quarters were hypoglycemic. After more coursework in human nutrition, I began to study the biochemistry of alcoholism in great depth. By 1981 I was ready to test the theories I had researched so carefully. I succeeded beyond my wildest imagination.

Today, alcoholism is the third leading cause of death in the United States. This book is dedicated to the many who did not recover and to those who have lost people they love to this terrible disease. It is addressed to those who have tried other forms of treatment and failed. Health Recovery Center's approach to treatment could very well have saved my son. It is too late for him, but it is not too late for you.

You will learn a lot about alcoholism in the chapters ahead, and you probably will also learn a lot about yourself. You will find some tests that will help you determine if you are alcoholic and what kind of alcoholic you are (yes, there are several types). You will learn why other treatment methods fail far more often than they succeed. I hope this information will inspire you to embark on this program with an open mind and an optimistic attitude. Too often alcoholics consider themselves failures and see their disease as a character flaw, rather than the illness it really is. Unfortunately, this attitude is all too common in our society. It adds to the pain alcoholics must endure when they realize that family members, friends, and even health professionals hold them responsible for their disease. Once you understand the biochemical disorders and changes that contribute to alcoholism, I hope you will be easier on yourself.

I suggest that you begin by reading this book straight through so you'll know what to expect when you begin the program. Then you can start at the beginning, take the tests, and use the book as a workbook to guide you through the program. Once you understand how profoundly alcohol can alter the chemistry of your body and brain, you'll be eager to begin the process of repair. You'll want to discover for yourself that it's possible to stop drinking without battling powerful cravings for alcohol. You'll want to change your diet to see if controlling hypoglycemic symptoms can actually make a difference in the way you feel. If depression is a problem for you, you'll want to try the treatments that can put it out of your life forever. However skeptical you may be now, I'm certain that what you are about to read will convince you that, at last, you've found the answers you've been seeking.

I know this program can work for you, but I urge you to follow it exactly as presented, one week at a time. At first glance, you may think that parts of it are a bit complex, but when you follow directions, you'll find that it is actually quite simple. I'll tell you exactly what to do and when to do it, what nutrients to take and when to take them. I have removed all the guesswork from this program, and each step has been carefully calculated to have maximum effect. That's why I must caution you to restrain your enthusiasm and curiosity. If you rush ahead too quickly, you'll lose many of the benefits. It undoubtedly took you much longer than seven weeks to conclude that you are alcoholic and longer still to admit that you need help. Seven weeks is not too long to invest in your recovery. The time will pass quickly because you'll start feeling better almost immediately. But I won't detain you any longer. Read on and begin your personal breakthrough to recovery from alcoholism.

Two

The Best-Kept Secret

- Craig had every reason to be depressed. He was drinking a quart of scotch a day, often without eating anything. Both his parents were alcoholic, and his father also suffered from severe depression. Craig was pale and thin. He had completed three alcoholism treatment programs, but nothing had succeeded in bringing his cravings under control. He was desperate for help.
- George, a burly young electrician, had been treated for alcoholism six times. Nothing worked. His parents had given up on him, and now his girlfriend threatened to leave him. When I first met him at ten o'clock in the morning, he smelled strongly of alcohol and spoke of suicide as the only way out of his misery.
- Alcoholism treatment counselors had expelled Sonnie from their program. Her bizarre behavior was driving them, and the other clients, crazy. The last straw came when Sonnie was found gig-

gling hilariously and painting zigzag lines on the walls of the basement furnace room. She had been assigned to paint the walls in exchange for treatment, work she had pledged to do because she couldn't afford to pay.

Craig, George, and Sonnie are all treatment failures. They are more the rule than the exception. The best-kept secret of alcoholism treatment today is that it doesn't work. Not for Craig, George, Sonnie and 75 percent of all those who check themselves in with high hopes for recovery.

Ironically, the blame for treatment failure is often placed on the patients. They're "not ready to stay sober" or "haven't reached bottom yet" say the counselors who staff these treatment programs. They assume that treatment works but patients fail. It is a curious perspective given the fact that most patients in treatment make an enormous commitment of time and money to be there. Doctors don't blame patients who are physically ill for failure to recover in response to treatment. They try another form of treatment, and another and another in an effort to effect a cure. Psychiatrists don't blame their mentally ill patients for failing to recover. They too try other forms of treatment.

This is not true of treatment for alcoholism. Despite acknowledged shortcomings, despite a shockingly high failure rate, there have been few innovations in the treatment of alcoholism in the past three decades. To understand this sad situation, you need to understand what treatment is available and why it so often misfires.

Treatment Programs

The Minnesota Model

Most alcoholism treatment in the United States today is a version of the Minnesota Model developed in the 1940s and 1950s by the Hazelden Foundation of Center City, Minnesota. This form of treatment is based on the presumption that drinking is a way of dealing with painful emotional or psychological problems and that once those problems are identified and confronted, the alcoholic will no longer be driven to drink irresponsibly. Typically, clients in treatment spend their days with counselors in group therapy. Everyone gets a chance to tell the story of how his life has become unmanageable because of alcoholism. Counselors and other members of the group help with the process of self-discovery by asking probing questions. The emotional release this process can trigger is thought to lower the need for compulsive drinking. The self-knowledge and insights gained about alcoholic behavior are believed to help alcoholics remain sober after treatment.

Most programs also require attendance at Alcoholics Anonymous meetings several times a week, if not daily.

Alcoholics Anonymous

Most people do not realize that Alcoholics Anonymous does not provide treatment. It is a support group, a fellowship through which alcoholics can become and remain abstinent with the help of other members. From the start, AA members acknowledge their powerlessness over alcohol. This acknowledgment is the first of the famous twelve steps (see page 14) members take toward spiritual awakening.

AA was founded in 1935 by Bill Wilson, a stockbroker, and Bob Smith, a physician, two alcoholics who helped each other to sobriety and then carried their message to others. Since then, AA has helped millions of alcoholics stop drinking. The organization keeps no statistics, but it is commonly reported that 25 to 30 percent of all members remain abstinent in their first year.

It is not widely known that before his death, Wilson was actively investigating the biochemical basis of alcoholism. When he died, his wife, Lois, wrote about his hopes to the researcher-physicians who were to carry on his work: her letter to Bill's psychiatrist friends was published in a pamphlet, *The Vitamin B-3 Therapy: A 3rd Communication to AA's Physicians.*

Aldous Huxley, a great admirer of A.A., introduced Bill to two psychiatrists who were researching the biochemistry of alcoholism . . . Bill was convinced of the truth of their findings and realized he could again help his beloved alcoholics by telling them about the physical component of alcoholism. As you know, Bill's

The Twelve Steps

1. We admitted we were powerless over alcohol—that our lives had become unmanageable.
2. Came to believe that a Power greater than ourselves could restore us to sanity.
3. Made a decision to turn our will and our lives over to the care of God as we understood Him.
4. Made a searching and fearless moral inventory of ourselves.
5. Admitted to God, to ourselves, and to another human being the exact nature of our wrongs.
6. Were entirely ready to have God remove all these defects of character.
7. Humbly asked Him to remove our shortcomings.
8. Made a list of all persons we had harmed, and became willing to make amends to them all.
9. Made direct amends to such people wherever possible, except when to do so would injure them or others.
10. Continued to take personal inventory and when we were wrong promptly admitted it.
11. Sought through prayer and meditation to improve our conscious contact with God as we understood Him, praying only for knowledge of His will for us and the power to carry that out.
12. Having had a spiritual awakening as the result of these Steps, we tried to carry this message to alcoholics, and to practice these principles in all our affairs.

Reprinted with permission of AA World Services, Inc.

last years were mainly devoted to the spread of this information among alcoholics and other ill persons. With your help, he wrote and distributed to A.A. doctors a brochure which has twice been enlarged and brought up to date . . . Bill's great hope was that continued research would find a means whereby those thousands of alcoholics who want to stop drinking but are too ill to grasp the

A.A. program could be released from their bondage and enabled to join A.A.

AA's approach is firmly entrenched in traditional treatment. Clients are often asked to take Step Four and "make a fearless and searching moral inventory of ourselves" and then to take Step Five and "admit to God, to ourselves and to another human being the exact nature of our wrongs."

Unfortunately, at this early stage of abstinence, many alcoholics simply aren't capable of this task. They're too damaged by alcohol to think clearly. These drinkers are the ones Bill W. worried about. They are too ill to benefit from AA.

A Dismal Success Rate

Take a look at Figure 1, which summarizes the results of 617 treatment follow-up studies. As you can see, even the most successful

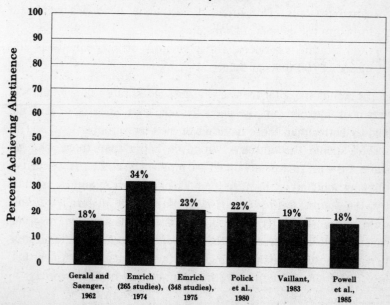

Figure 1. Abstinence Achieved Through Conventional Treatment: Results of 617 Follow-up Studies

programs did not help even half of their clients remain sober for one to two years. Only 24 percent of those treated managed to stay away from alcohol for two years.

Ironically, studies of alcoholics who stopped drinking without treatment have produced almost identical results. A fascinating study at the Kansas City Veterans Administration Medical Center demonstrated what can be expected from different approaches to treatment. The researchers compared three groups of alcoholics:

- Those who got no treatment at all beyond a fifteen-minute medical appointment once a month
- Those who received Antabuse, a drug that makes you sick when you drink alcohol
- Those who got a full range of treatment services, including an outpatient treatment program, family counseling, individual counseling and therapy, vocational and rehabilitation guidance, AA, and the option of taking Antabuse

At the end of one year, here's how the three groups compared:

- No treatment: Thirty-seven of the fifty alcoholics were still drinking (76 percent failure rate)
- Antabuse only: Thirty-nine of forty-nine alcoholics were still drinking (80 percent failure rate)
- Full treatment services: Thirty-nine out of forty-nine were still drinking (80 percent failure rate)

The results speak for themselves: the success rate (22 percent) was very poor. Inexplicably, the alcoholics who got no treatment at all did slightly better than those in either of the other groups.

Why should the untreated group do better than those who got state-of-the-art treatment? Could the problem lie at the root of current thinking about alcoholism? In the bible of modern American psychiatry, the *Diagnostic and Statistical Manual of Mental Disorders,* third edition (DSM-III), alcoholism is classified as a *mental* disorder. Almost exclusively, treatment consists of talk: counseling, confrontation. And despite the depressingly high percentage of treatment failure (and counselor burnout), the approach has never wavered.

Alcoholism and Health

It is no secret that alcoholism takes a terrible toll on physical health. A 1989 report in *Alcohol World,* a publication of the National Institute on Alcohol Abuse and Alcoholism, an average of twenty years of life is lost by alcoholics, who generally die before age sixty-five from alcohol-related causes. Cirrhosis of the liver is the primary killer, but heavy drinking is also associated with heart disease and several types of cancer. Tragically, some alcoholics don't even live long enough to get most of these terrible diseases. Among young alcoholics, the death rates from suicide, accidents, and cirrhosis are ten times higher than normal.

Less well known is the fact that the death rate among recovered alcoholics is almost as high as it is among those who continue to drink. This surprising—and disappointing—finding emerged from a five-year study of a group of alcoholic employees of the Du Pont company. Some of the alcoholics continued to drink, but about one-third were abstinent. The group was compared to an equal number of nonalcoholics of the same age, sex, and payroll class. At the end of the five years, the death rate among the alcoholics was almost 12 percent, compared to 3.7 percent among the nonalcoholics. And when the researchers compared the abstinent alcoholics to those who continued to drink, they found only a slight difference in the death rate, which was 3.6 times higher than normal among the drinkers and 2.9 times higher among the recovered alcoholics.

Can the high death rate among the treated alcoholics be prevented? Unfortunately, this issue has not been addressed in conventional treatment programs, and in the research I reviewed, I found no strategies aimed at halting physical deterioration and reducing early mortality among recovered alcoholics. Clearly, new methods are needed to treat the physical damage from alcohol that causes early death.

Alcohol and the Mind

After my son's death, I believed that everyone else in treatment was recovering successfully and that Rob's suicide was an isolated occurrence. I discovered how wrong I was. The shocking truth emerged in 1984, nine years after Rob died: one in four deaths among treated alcoholics is a suicide. Most of these suicides take place in the first year after treatment.

Now I know that depression severe enough to lead to suicide is common among abstinent alcoholics and that many never regain a feeling of emotional well-being. This was brought home to me forcefully one evening not long after Health Recovery Center was founded. At a reception in another city, I was introduced to a man who had just received his twenty-five-year AA medallion for successful sobriety. He was one of a group who had attended a meeting at which I explained my concept of treatment for alcoholism. Later that evening, he took me aside and confided that after all those years he still fought intense cravings for alcohol and fantasized about one last wonderful drinking binge after which he would drive his car into an abutment. I was stunned to hear that he was still struggling with such demons. I offered him treatment at HRC, but he turned me down.

I wish I could tell you that this man represents only a minority of abstinent alcoholics and that most are emotionally stable and have rediscovered a positive sense of purpose and a zest for life. I have searched and searched in vain for studies to confirm this, but I have found just the opposite. A vast number of abstinent alcoholics continue to battle depression and crave alcohol, never regaining lost territory in their personal lives and careers. Alcoholism casts a long, dark shadow on their lives for years after they quit drinking.

What Time Doesn't Heal

For the majority of alcoholics, abstinence is not all it's cracked up to be. In 1962, a team of psychiatrists studied 299 alcoholics who had completed treatment at six different centers and reported how they were faring one year later (D. Gerard and S. Saenger, "The Abstinent Alcoholic," *Archives of General Psychiatry*). Sadly, 82 percent had resumed drinking. But the picture wasn't much rosier for the fifty-five who remained abstinent:

- Fifty-four percent were "overtly disturbed," which, the researchers explained, meant that their abstinence was "sustained in context of an unstable state; they suffer with tension to a degree which concerns them; they are angry, driven by anxiety, restless, unable to relax, seek to distract themselves by spending inordinate amounts of time at work or in social activities of a community nature; and/or are overtly psychiatrically ill displaying disturbances of mood, thought and behavior to a psychotic degree."
- Twenty-four percent were classified as "inconspicuously inadequate: meagerness of involvement with life; no positive sense of excitement, purpose or interest in life."
- Twelve percent were deemed AA successes, having "acquired a sense of purpose and value in life through their AA membership. It is evident that they are as dependent on AA as they were before on alcohol and the patterns of relationships in which their alcoholism was integrated."
- Ten percent were rated "independent successes in that they do not appear disturbed, are more alive and interesting as human beings, engage in a variety of personal interactions on the basis of positive interest; efforts at self-realization are independent rather than institutionally supported."

In conclusion, the researchers commented that they were "astonished to note how prolonged abstinence could accompany gross mental disturbances and maladjustments."

Ten Years Later

As the case of the twenty-five-year AA veteran illustrates, time does not necessarily heal the consequences of alcoholism. When alcoholics first stop drinking, they are led to believe that they will soon be feeling good. For most, that doesn't happen—their anxiety and depression will be with them for many years. Results of a ten-year study by researchers at Johns Hopkins University (C. De Soto et al.) demon-

strated that the typical alcoholic experiences most of the following
symptoms for years into recovery:

- Depression
- Anxiety
- Psychosis (lack of contact with reality)
- Hostility
- Feelings of inadequacy and inferiority
- Paranoia
- Phobic anxiety

The researchers reported that the intensity of these symptoms
diminished slowly over time; by the tenth year, many of the 312
alcoholics participating in the study showed significant improvement.

Given the grim outlook, it isn't surprising that so many alcoholics
resume drinking. When sobriety doesn't deliver on its promise to ease
their suffering, they opt for a quicker fix—alcohol. Can we blame
them? It's human nature to seek relief from stress. Few of us would
do much better.

Relapse Is the Norm

Relapse among treated alcoholics is so prevalent that professional
journals label one-year follow-up studies of treatment outcome as
"long term." The extent of the relapse problem was demonstrated in
1980 in the Rand Report, the results of a federally funded four-year
study of 922 alcoholic men who had been treated in seven hospitals.
Here's what the research team found:

- Of the 922 men, only 28 percent refrained from drinking for six
  months after treatment
- After one year, only 21 percent remained abstinent
- After four years, only 7 percent remained abstinent

My educated guess is that the abstinent 7 percent have spent most
of their four years involved with support or therapy groups, using AA
or psychotherapy to "adjust" their attitudes and "manage" their unstable emotions.

Among professionals in the field, the fact that treatment doesn't work well is an open secret. No less an authority than Enoch Gordis, M.D., director of the National Institute on Alcohol Abuse and Alcoholism, has conceded this publicly: "The treatment of alcoholism has not improved in any important way in twenty-five years . . . Only a minority of patients who enter treatment are helped to long-term recovery."

Teaching Alcoholics to Drink Socially

The presumption that alcoholism stems from an underlying emotional disorder reasonably suggests that once the "problem" is uncovered and dealt with in therapy, alcoholics should be able to drink moderately like everybody else. Every chapter of AA has members who have tested or are testing this theory without success.

Researchers have also attempted to show that alcoholics can be taught to drink moderately. In 1973, California psychologists Mark and Linda Sobell reported on a study in which they used behavior-modification techniques to train twenty alcoholic men as social drinkers. The Sobells had followed the men for two years and reported that 85 percent were "drinking moderately or not at all." The results made headlines nationwide. And why not? They contradicted established AA wisdom and suggested that alcoholism was a psychological disorder that could be treated and cured with behavioral therapy.

The trouble is, it wasn't true.

Ten years later, another team of researchers decided to take a second look at how the twenty men were doing. Their findings were shocking. Nineteen of the twenty men *never* drank moderately; the other subject had been mistakenly classified as an alcoholic and shouldn't have been in the study. Contrary to the Sobells' claims, records showed that most of the men had been rehospitalized for alcoholism treatment within one year of discharge from the research project. Today, four are dead from suicide and other alcohol-related causes, and nine continued drinking, their lives in shambles. Only six managed to become abstinent with treatment and the aid of AA.

The harm that the Sobells' widely publicized study caused cannot be measured. For ten years, many alcoholics believed the distorted results and tried to become social drinkers. Even now, most alcoholics want to believe that controlled drinking is possible. But research tells us otherwise. In 1985, the prestigious *New England Journal of Medicine* published results of a study of 1,239 alcoholics who had completed hospital-based treatment programs. The researchers had followed the group for five to seven years and found that *less than 2 percent were able to drink alcohol without losing control.* The researchers also found that 79 percent of the alcoholics who survived were drinking heavily at the time of follow-up. Only 7 percent had stopped drinking; 14 percent were dead. One participating hospital reported an appalling 45 percent mortality rate among alcoholic study subjects within the five- to seven-year span of the study. The researchers concluded that there is "little cause for optimism about the likelihood of an evolution to long-term, stable, moderate drinking among alcoholics."

Putting It All Together

My search for answers to Rob's suicide led me through most of the current research about alcoholism and how it is treated today. Certain facts emerged repeatedly:

- Current treatment emphasizes behavioral and psychological rehabilitation based on the assumption that emotional and/or sociological problems trigger heavy drinking
- Psychologists and psychiatrists working in the field describe alcoholism as a mental disorder and attempt to treat it as such
- Despite the variety of therapies available in treatment settings, recovery rates are consistently poor; relapse is the norm
- Present treatment methods fail to relieve depression and anxiety, end alcoholic cravings, or help alcoholics overcome unstable moods
- Whether alcoholics recover on their own or with treatment, only about 25 percent sustain some abstinence
- One in four deaths among treated alcoholics is due to suicide

- The mortality rate among both treated and untreated alcoholics is about three times higher than among the general population

It's a bleak picture, and a puzzling one. In science, when a theory is tested and fails to deliver on its promise, it is deemed disproved, a null hypothesis. At that point, researchers know they must discard the faulty hypothesis and search for a new answer. In scientific terminology, clinging to a disproven theory is an error of the first kind. Data from studies of alcoholism treatment have demonstrated again and again that we are locked into this kind of major error in our concept of alcoholism as a psychological disorder. Present methods have been failing us. Most alcoholics do not recover. Ultimately, they die of this disease. It is time to relinquish old beliefs and search for new answers.

A New Direction

The more I learned about alcoholism, the more I became convinced that it is not just a psychological disorder or a sign of emotional weakness or flawed character that can be resolved with talk therapy. Instead, I began to see alcoholism as a physical disease, the outcome of a powerful physical addiction to alcohol that gradually inflicts mortal damage to brain and body chemistry. The ample and growing evidence of its genetic underpinnings convinced me that only certain people were vulnerable to this addiction. I found support for my views in some surprising quarters.

William Mayer, M.D., former chief of the U.S. Alcohol, Drug Abuse, and Mental Health Administration, speaks of alcoholism as "a disease . . . genetically determined . . . clearly progressive. We can predict its course even though the speed of its course may vary from person to person. It is ultimately fatal. It leads to a predictable physical deterioration and often some mental impairment, and it occurs in people who have *no discernible previous psychological or emotional disorders*" (italics mine).

In 1982, the question of whether alcoholism is a physical or mental disorder was the subject of a major courtroom battle. The case pitted the federal government against Granville House, an alcoholism treatment center in Minneapolis that treats many uninsured clients who receive government disability funding. The government's position was that since alcoholism was classified officially as a mental disorder, Medicare could rightly refuse to reimburse Granville House for the treatment it provided.

The government's star witness was a psychiatrist, Dr. Robert Spitzer, who defended the view of alcoholism as a psychological disorder even though he recognized that "there exists no effective psychiatric treatment."

Two former presidents of the American Society of Addiction Medicine—LeClair Bissell, M.D., and Maxwell Weisman, M.D.—testified in support of the concept of alcoholism as a physiological disease. In summing up their testimony, federal judge Miles Lord noted that they had described "the utter failure of treatment modalities based on defining, diagnosing, and treating alcoholism as a mental disease."

In his decision, Judge Lord noted that the American Medical Association had classified alcoholism as a physical disease in 1957. Here is an excerpt from his opinion:

> Alcoholism is the third leading cause of death in the United States. This Court is unaware of any mental illness that so directly and persistently results in death . . . Disease of the body, if severe and continuing, will in time affect the mind . . . The sole fact that a condition is accompanied by abnormal behavior does not justify its classification as mental. The great bulk of the testimony supports the conclusion that alcoholism is a diagnosis of a primary disease. It cannot be understood as a secondary effect of any other problems. The disease is predominantly physical as opposed to mental in nature . . . It is therefore the Court's conclusion that the Federal Government's classification of alcoholism and other forms of chemical dependency as mental disorders is arbitrary and capricious.

So far, this decision and the long-standing position of the AMA and the World Health Organization have had little impact on treatment for alcoholism. Psychological talk therapy continues to prevail.

Old Questions, New Answers

Despite the enormous body of research showing the frightening toll alcohol takes on the body and the brain, the question of what might be done to repair the damage remains unasked and unanswered. As I read through all the studies documenting the damage caused by heavy drinking, I kept thinking, What if? What if we did more than counsel alcoholics? What if rehabilitation consisted of more than just talk therapy?

Most of my questions related to Rob's death.

Q. How could a normal kid who loved life become so depressed that he committed suicide?

A. Rob had shown no signs of depression before he began drinking. The alcohol must have altered his brain chemistry to cause the hopeless depression that precipitated his suicide.

Q. Why couldn't the therapy and emotional support he received in treatment and at AA restore him to his old self?

A. The damage to his brain and nervous system couldn't be talked away.

Q. What could have been done to cure his depression?

A. A number of brain chemicals known to prevent depression are depleted by heavy drinking. Was there a way to restore them? Could hypoglycemia have contributed to Rob's depression? Depletion of certain nutrients has been linked to depression. Lab testing might have provided clues to what imbalances had developed and what could be done to restore him to normal.

Q. If disorders of body and brain chemistry detected in lab tests could be corrected, would he have been able to recover?

That is the $64,000 question. To answer it I needed to develop a system for biological repair. I had read hundreds of research papers that described the functions of our brain and body chemicals and the symptoms that develop when they are depleted. There were hundreds of other papers that described the effect of alcoholism on these natural chemicals. Together, this research suggested a scientific basis for a new approach to treatment that combines biochemical repair with counseling and the support of Alcoholics Anonymous.

At the outset I knew there would be resistance to this approach. The notion that the roots of alcoholism are in body chemistry is not easy to accept. My theory that it might be possible to fix what had been broken was, at that point, an educated guess that was met with great skepticism.

But I persisted, and the answers I sought after Rob's death led to a treatment model that has proven far more effective than I dared dream. Today, there *is* a way to overcome addictive cravings, depression, and the many other alcohol-induced symptoms that trigger relapse. The pages that follow will guide you to recovery, a gift to you from Rob.

Three

It's Not All in Your Mind

Alcoholism runs in families. Even before researchers showed how and why some people are predisposed to becoming alcoholic, simple observation showed that when one or both parents are alcoholic, the children are at risk. Until recently, researchers couldn't be sure whether this familial link was hereditary or environmental or both. Do people drink because they "learned to" at home, or do they drink because they are genetically programmed to become alcoholic? While the environmental influence certainly can't be discounted, new evidence strongly suggests that heredity plays a much stronger role in alcoholism than was once thought.

What Twins Can Tell Us

Much of the new evidence comes from comparisons of identical and fraternal twins. Since identical twins develop from a single fertilized egg that divides after conception, both have the exact same genetic makeup and can be expected to be alike in most respects. For example, identical twins are always the same sex, always have the same hair and eye color, and usually reach the same adult height and weight. Studies of identical twins separated at birth and raised in different families have produced compelling evidence of the power of their genetic bond. In addition to their strikingly similar physical development, the twins have remarkably similar tastes, preferences, and interests.

Fraternal twins develop from two different eggs fertilized by two different sperm. Fraternal twins are no more closely related than siblings born separately.

If environment were the sole cause of alcoholism, the rate of alcoholism among twins raised in drinking families should be the same regardless of whether they are identical or fraternal. But if a genetic predisposition were responsible, the rate of alcoholism would be similar among both identical twins, who have exactly the same genes. Studies have shown that when one identical twin is alcoholic, the other is four times more likely to be alcoholic than when one fraternal twin is alcoholic, indicating that genetics play a part in alcoholism.

There have been many other studies aimed at showing whether nature or nurture is to blame for alcoholism. One of the first (Donald Goodwin, 1973) compared 133 sons of alcoholics adopted and raised by nonalcoholic parents to a similar group of adoptees with no genetic history of alcoholism. The sons of alcoholics were three times more likely to become alcoholic than the sons of nonalcoholic parents. A larger study in Sweden (C. R. Cloninger, M. Bohman, and S. Sigvardsson, 1981) followed 3,000 adoptees separated from their biological parents at an early age and raised by nonrelatives. The risk of these children becoming alcoholic was two and a half times higher when one biological parent was alcoholic.

Researchers have also studied what happens to the children of nonalcoholics who are adopted into households where one parent is alcoholic. They have found no evidence that being raised by an alcoholic parent predisposes a child to alcoholism.

Under the Microscope

Research indicates that some hereditary abnormality of body or brain chemistry must be passed from generation to generation to account for the fact that alcoholism runs in families. The search for such an abnormality has yielded a number of valuable clues. The first was the discovery of certain unusual brain-wave patterns among alcoholics and their nondrinking children. P3 brain waves, which influence memory, were absent or weaker than normal among the alcoholic families studied. (Not coincidentally, memory lapses are common complaints among alcoholics.)

Researchers discovered that alcoholics are much more likely than nonalcoholics to have a certain gene affecting receptor sites for dopamine, a central-nervous-system neurotransmitter that facilitates communication between nerve cells and is associated with pleasure-seeking behavior. Researchers theorize that the newly discovered gene alters dopamine receptor sites in the brain. Receptor sites can be thought of as locks that can be opened only by the correct chemical key—in this case, dopamine. Exactly how the new gene predisposes a person to alcoholism isn't yet known, but the fact that it was found in 77 percent of the alcoholics studied and was absent in 72 percent of nonalcoholics suggests that it underlies some types of alcoholism.

More Chemical Clues

Discoveries about the way alcohol is processed in the body have provided further evidence of a genetic link. For example, Harvard scientists (L. Tunglai et al., 1977) recently came upon a previously unknown liver enzyme responsible for metabolizing alcohol. This enzyme, alcohol dehydrogenase II (II ADH), can process or oxidize alcohol up to 40 percent more efficiently than the liver enzymes most

of us have. People who have this enzyme—and most of us do not—
have an inborn ability to drink very large amounts of alcohol without
becoming intoxicated. These are the folks who can drink many of us
under the table without getting the least bit tipsy and or feeling hung
over the next morning.

Researchers have also discovered that the absence of a crucial liver
enzyme accounts for the fact that very few Orientals become alcoholics. In fact, many Asians get sick whenever they drink. Their pulses
race and they feel dizzy and nauseated. The explanation for this
peculiar reaction is the fact that many Orientals have only one liver
enzyme that processes alcohol, rather than the two found in people
from other parts of the world. About half the Oriental population is
missing this second crucial enzyme.

Alcoholics and nonalcoholics process alcohol differently. When alcohol reaches the liver, it is changed into acetaldehyde, a harmful
byproduct of alcohol metabolism that can damage liver cells. Normally, the liver rapidly transforms the harmful acetaldehyde into a
neutral substance called acetic acid or acetate. The acetic acid is then
converted into carbon dioxide and water. We expel the carbon dioxide
through respiration and the water through urination.

Until recently, it was believed that the liver always handles alcohol
in the same way. But new research shows that a different scenario
occurs among certain alcoholics and children of alcoholics with no
drinking experience (Figure 2). Their livers change alcohol into acetaldehyde at twice the normal rate, while the subsequent conversion
of acetaldehyde into acetic acid is abnormally slow and takes twice as
long as usual. The accumulation of acetaldehyde damages liver cells,
which become abnormally large as they strive to get rid of the accumulated acetaldehyde. This damage affects the liver's ability to
absorb and utilize the nutrients needed for good health. To make
matters worse, excess acetaldehyde escapes the liver and travels
through the bloodstream to the heart, where it can be very damaging
(it interferes with the protein synthesis of the heart muscle). It also
reaches the brain, where it blocks proper neurotransmitter action in
creating normal feelings, behavior, and memory. The unused natural
neurotransmitters begin to build up and combine with the acetaldehyde to form potent psychoactive compounds called tetrahy-

Figure 2. How the Body Breaks Down Alcohol

Alcoholic Chemistry	Nonalcoholic Chemistry

Alcohol

Changes twice as rapidly to acetaldehyde

↓

Acetaldehyde

Inhibits heart protein synthesis

Combines with brain neurotransmitters to make tetrahydroisoquinolines (THIQs) (addictive and euphoric morphine-like substances)

Acetic Acid

CO_2
Carbon dioxide (leaves via lungs)

H_2O
Water (leaves via kidneys)

Alcohol

↓

Acetaldehyde

Changes twice as rapidly to acetic acid

Acetic Acid

CO_2
Carbon dioxide (leaves via lungs)

H_2O
Water (leaves via kidneys)

droisoquinolines (THIQs), which are remarkably similar to opiates. THIQs fit in the same receptor sites in the brain as natural pain-killing chemicals called endorphins and such narcotics as morphine and heroin.

The Chemistry of Addiction

Two decades ago, Texas researcher Virginia Davis noticed during autopsies of skid row alcoholics that their brains contained an opiate that she first mistook for heroin. This was puzzling because these indigents did not have the money needed to support such an expensive drug habit. The heroin-like substance turned out to be THIQs that had been manufactured inside their brains when acetaldehyde from the breakdown of alcohol had combined with natural neurotransmitters. Davis's data support the concept of alcoholism as a true addiction stemming from specific biochemical events leading to the formation of an addictive substance similar to opiates such as heroin.

We now know that in heavy drinkers, THIQs displace endorphins and bind with the opiate receptors in the brain. In doing so, they signal the brain to stop producing endorphins. As the natural endorphin supply declines, more and more alcohol is needed to produce more THIQs to replace the natural endorphins and bind with opiate receptors to create feelings of well-being.

At the University of Texas, researcher Kenneth Blum, M.D., found that restoring these natural endorphins and neurotransmitters destroyed or depleted by alcohol will reduce cravings for alcohol and restore normal moods.

Some pertinent findings emerged from a study of the reactions to alcohol among two groups of college students. One group was composed of students who had a family history of alcoholism; those in the second group had no alcoholism in their backgrounds. After four drinks, the students from alcoholic families produced much higher levels of acetaldehyde, and they could perform a variety of mental and physical tests *better* under the influence of four drinks than when they had not been drinking. The students with no family history of alcoholism reported feeling moderately intoxicated and showed impaired physical dexterity, reflexes, mental ability after four drinks.

Allergic/Addicted:
Same Diagnosis, Different Chemistry

Not all alcoholics fit neatly into the pattern described above. Some may actually be allergic to alcohol. This theory has been advanced by Theron Randolph, M.D., the father of clinical ecology, a new field of medicine that contends that allergies to foods and environmental chemicals cause a number of physical conditions. Randolph has shown that addictions to food and alcohol can produce alternating highs and lows. The highs are feelings of well-being that occur when the body is supplied with the addictive substance; the lows are withdrawal symptoms. In his work with members of Alcoholics Anonymous, Randolph discovered that many were allergic/addicted to the sugars, grapes, and grains from which alcohol is made. He demonstrated that these people begin to crave alcohol when exposed to the underlying component to which they are addicted. In addition to Randolph's work, a study of 422 alcoholics by an Illinois researcher, Herbert Karolus, M.D., showed that most were allergic to wheat or rye, the grain bases of many distilled liquors.

An allergic response can affect any organ in the body. The skin may react with hives, the intestinal tract with diarrhea, the brain with migraine headaches or altered moods and behavior. Alcohol can wreak havoc on the brain chemistry of allergic/addicted individuals. Their first drinking experience is always unpleasant. Their bodies send a clear message of alcohol intolerance by making them feel ill. Unfortunately, many people try to overcome this and "learn to drink." With repeated doses of alcohol, their bodies have no choice but to adapt. Allergist William Philpott, M.D., describes this adaptation as an allergic/addicted response to alcohol. The pattern begins with a high when alcohol is ingested. One of the ways the body reacts to substances to which it is allergic is by producing its own addictive narcotics, the opioid endorphins, which create a feeling of euphoria. Once the pleasurable endorphin effect, the high, wears off, the withdrawal phase occurs. This is often manifested by emotional symptoms: depression, confusion, anxiety. The only way to overcome these feelings is with another dose of the addictive substance.

In the early stages of this type of alcoholism, drinking provides only a gentle lift. The equally subtle letdown that comes later is usually not associated with the pleasure of drinking. But in time, the period of pleasure becomes shorter, while the withdrawal symptoms become more intense.

Given this pattern, it is easy to understand why the allergic drinker returns to alcohol in an effort to avoid the pain of withdrawal. Unlike the II ADH/THIQ alcoholic, who can tolerate large amounts of alcohol with minimal behavioral changes and mild or no hangovers, the allergic/addicted alcoholic tends to be a binge drinker who loses control easily. People with this kind of chemistry typically get hangovers.

They also have a tendency, when drinking, toward altered personality: sudden anger, depression, or abusiveness caused by the allergic response of their brains and central nervous systems.

Environmental Culprits

Clinical ecologists have also found that exposure to such toxic chemicals as gasoline, cleaning solvents, and formaldehyde can cause alcoholic cravings in sensitive individuals. If they inhale fumes from these chemicals on a daily basis, the same allergic/addicted adaptive mechanism described above can occur. These people can become mildly intoxicated as a result of breathing the fumes from such chemicals. They often find that they can maintain the high and ward off the letdown by heading for the bar at the end of the workday.

Take the case of Janet, a single parent, who cleaned offices at night. She sought our help for her intense depression. Janet had recently joined AA and was no longer drinking, but she still craved alcohol and battled suicidal thoughts. Driving home from work early one morning, she had to fight a powerful compulsion to steer her car over a bridge or into a tree.

Janet's work exposed her daily to fumes from a number of cleaning solvents. We sent her for tests to determine if the chemicals she was inhaling at work played any role in her depression and craving for alcohol. When tested for sensitivity to ethanol (alcohol), she first felt high, almost intoxicated, then became withdrawn, and finally burst into tears and cried uncontrollably. Ethanol in any form (alcohol, cleaning fluids, gasoline, perfume) was the root of Janet's problem. After she found a job that no longer exposed her to ethanol fumes, she recovered quickly. Both her cravings and her depression vanished.

Common environmental chemicals not only set the stage for alcoholism, they can also precipitate relapse, as they have in many alcoholics whose AA peers unfairly labeled them "weak" or "not working their program." In such people, uncontrollable cravings for alcohol can be turned on by provocative testing in clinical-ecology laboratories. Once activated, these cravings are powerful enough to overcome the strongest defenses against alcohol. Their effect on the brain robs sensitive individuals of the ability to make responsible decisions.

A Family Affair:
Essential Fatty Acids

More chemical clues to the nature of alcoholism come from research focusing on alcoholics with at least one grandparent who was Welsh, Irish, Scottish, Scandinavian, or native American. Typically, these alcoholics have a history of depression going back to childhood and close relatives who suffered from depression or schizophrenia. Some may have relatives who committed suicide. There also may be a family history of eczema, cystic fibrosis, premenstrual syndrome, diabetes, irritable bowel syndrome, or benign breast disease.

The common denominator here is a genetic abnormality in the way the body handles certain essential fatty acids (EFAs) derived from foods. Normally, these EFAs are converted in the brain to various metabolites such as prostaglandin E_1 (PGE_1), which plays a vital role in the prevention of depression, convulsions, and hyperexcitability. When the EFA conversion process is defective, brain levels of prostaglandin E_1 are lower than normal, which results in depression.

In affected individuals, alcohol acts as a double-edged sword. It activates the PGE_1 within the brain, which immediately lifts depression and creates feelings of well-being. Because the brain cannot make new PGE_1 efficiently, its meager supply of PGE_1 is gradually depleted. Over time, the ability of alcohol to lift depression slowly diminishes.

Several years ago, researchers hit upon a solution to this problem. They discovered that a natural substance, oil of evening primrose, contains large amounts of gamma-linolenic acid (GLA), which can help the brain convert EFAs to PGE_1.

The results are quite dramatic. In a recent study in Scotland, researcher David Horrobin, M.D., matched two groups of alcoholics whose EFA levels were 50 percent below normal. The first group got EFA replacement, the second, a placebo. Marked differences between the two groups emerged in the withdrawal stage. The group that got EFA replacement had far fewer symptoms, while the placebo group displayed the full range of withdrawal symptoms associated with prostaglandin deficiency: tremors, irritability, tension, hyperexcitability, and convulsions.

At the outset of the study, members of both groups had some degree of alcohol-related liver damage. Three months later, the researchers found that liver function among the EFA replacement group was almost normal. There was no significant improvement among the placebo group.

A year later, the placebo group was still deficient in the natural ability to convert essential fatty acids into PGE_1. What's more, only 28 percent of this group had remained sober; the rest had resumed drinking. Results were dramatically better among the EFA replacement group: 83 percent remained sober and depression free.

Is There an Alcoholic Personality?

One of the most persistent myths about alcoholism is that it stems from some sort of personality disorder. Dr. George Vaillant, an eminent Harvard psychiatrist, has spent forty years trying to determine if there is any truth to this popular conception. His team of psychologists and sociologists has studied more than 650 young men in hopes of finding traits that predict alcoholism. In a 1984 report on his long-term study, Vaillant concluded that there is no evidence to support the belief that personality disorders predispose a person to alcoholism:

> Future alcoholics do NOT appear different from future asymptomatic drinkers in terms of premorbid psychological stability. It is the heavy use of alcohol which causes personality alternations.
>
> Even sociopathic behavior is almost always a consequence, not a cause of alcohol abuse.
>
> Just as light passing through water confounds our perceptions, the illness of alcoholism profoundly distorts the individual's personality.

For a better understanding of Dr. Vaillant's conclusions, let's take a look at one of his subjects, James O'Neill, chosen for the study at age nineteen. This case study is taken from Dr. Vaillant's book *The Natural History of Alcoholism*.

Vaillant's study group was composed of college sophomores chosen on the basis of their psychological health. At the time, in the forties, the dean's office rated O'Neill's stability as A and ranked him in the top third of the study group. The project psychiatrist described O'Neill's parents as "reliable, consistent, obsessive" and devoted. O'Neill's relationship with his mother was rated among the best in the study. In 1950, six months after his mother died, O'Neill still felt the loss deeply.

When he was twenty-one, O'Neill married his high school girlfriend, whom he had been in love with since age sixteen. Six years later the marriage still seemed solid.

O'Neill had begun drinking heavily in 1948, and by 1950 he had begun drinking in the morning. He admitted that between 1952 and 1955 he had written his Ph.D. dissertation while continuously intoxicated and had regularly sold books from the university library in order to support his drinking. By 1955, his alcoholism was campus gossip; by 1957, O'Neill recognized that his pattern of drinking, sexual infidelity, gambling, and unrepaid borrowing suggested a psychopathic personality. In discussions with a psychologist in the 1960s, O'Neill voiced no sorrow about his mother's death and could not even remember when she had died. Later, a psychiatrist observed that O'Neill "felt quite hostile and anxious about the fact that he was an army brat and never had a normal childhood, and his parents were always very cold toward him. He harbored many feelings of hostility toward his wife."

In 1970, when he was fifty-two, O'Neill stopped drinking and joined AA. Two years later he described himself to a project psychiatrist as "a classic psychopath totally incapable of commitment to any man alive . . . I'm hyperemotional . . . In AA, I'm known as Dr. Anti-Serenity."

What happened to this promising, psychologically stable young man?

There is no doubt that his brain no longer served him normally. His thinking had become negative. He felt isolated and hyperactive. A reasonable explanation for his personality changes is that heavy alcohol use gradually disrupted his normal brain function by blocking or destroying the natural chemicals that maintain emotional stability. This kind of chemical disruption cannot be talked away by therapy.

Your Alcoholic Brain: The Malfunctioning Computer

Recent discoveries about the workings of the brain have shed important new light on the role a wide variety of natural chemicals play in maintaining normal thought patterns, feelings, self-awareness, memory, and perception. There is also an enormous body of research to show that alcohol diminishes or destroys many of the substances the brain must use to create and regulate our emotions. The human mind cannot operate in a vacuum. It depends on the molecular functioning of the brain to maintain mental processes and emotional health.

For the parents, husbands, wives, and friends of an alcoholic, there is some comfort in knowing that the personality changes they have observed are a result of alterations in normal brain chemistry caused by heavy drinking. It is no more logical to blame the alcoholic for altered behavior than to demand accountability from someone with Alzheimer's disease. They don't choose to behave as they do. They are ill, victims of chemical changes they cannot control.

My search for an explanation for my son's suicide finally ended when I came to understand how alcohol had affected his brain, altered his personality, and turned him into a suicidally depressed young man.

But this understanding gave rise to more questions. What could be done to prevent similar tragedies? Is there no way to undo the damage alcohol causes?

As I pondered these questions, I began to wonder about the value of the conventional approach to the treatment of alcoholism. For all the spiritual resources provided by AA and the psychological insights available in counseling and group therapy, no attempts were being made to undo the damaging effects of alcohol on the delicate chemical balance that keeps the brain and central nervous system functioning normally. Why weren't we trying to fix what alcohol had broken?

Was I overlooking something? Surely others had asked the same questions that nagged at me. George Vaillant had brilliantly and conclusively demonstrated that the alcoholic's unstable behavior is a consequence, not a cause, of alcoholism and that personality changes stem from the physical damage done by this disease. Was there no treatment to repair that damage?

Back to the Drawing Board

In 1896 Sigmund Freud predicted that "the future may teach us to exercise a direct influence by means of chemical substances upon the amounts of energy and their distribution in the apparatus of the mind." By 1927 he had become "firmly convinced that one day all these mental disturbances we are trying to understand will be treated by means of hormones or similar substances."

Today, we see how right he was. We now have drugs to treat depression, the schizophrenias, and obsessive-compulsive disorder. And lying unused in libraries everywhere are reports on studies of the destructive effect of alcohol on the mind and body through its power to inhibit access to key amino acids, vitamins, minerals, trace elements, enzymes, hormones, and essential fatty acids—the natural chemicals that support life and sustain sanity.

My question was whether it would be possible to restore depleted or damaged natural chemicals. If it was, I theorized, recovery from alcoholism might be more successful than it was with current treatment.

Nobel Prize laureate Linus Pauling coined the word "orthomolecular" to describe the process of "establishing the right molecules in the body by varying the concentrations of substances normally present and required for optimum health." Could orthomolecular treatment be the answer I sought? At the time I had been working as a chemical-dependency counselor for five years and was weary of seeing people discharged when they were still depressed and ill. My peers didn't see what I was getting at. Small wonder; their training hadn't included the study of the physical basis of psychological problems.

But the clients understood. They were painfully aware that therapy had failed to eliminate their cravings, anxiety, insomnia, depression, and mental confusion. I finally decided to test my theories to see what would happen by combining biochemical repair with traditional treatment for alcoholism. In January 1981 I established the Health Recovery Center as a pilot program offering physical detoxification and biochemical repair along with counseling and participation in Alcoholics Anonymous.

We focused on the internal symptoms as well as the obvious external calamities that brought our clients to treatment. We knew they could put their calamities behind them, but it would take more than talk to relieve the agony emanating from their chemically disrupted brains.

Biochemical Repair

Our biochemical repair program is built around two premises:

1. Addressing the substances that must be kept out of the alcoholic's body (including alcohol and other drugs, such as nicotine, caffeine, and refined sugars)
2. Addressing the substances that must be restored (brain and body chemicals depleted by alcohol)

We begin with a physical exam and laboratory testing to identify where damage has occurred. Clients are also screened for vulnerability to substances that can cause cravings for alcohol.

At the outset we explain why it's so important that clients avoid caffeine, nicotine, and refined sugars in addition to alcohol. We were amazed at how much coffee our clients had been drinking; some were up to forty cups a day. Caffeine is a drug. Although it recently received a clean bill of health for those concerned about heart disease and cancer, it can complicate or retard recovery from alcoholism. Caffeine pumps a lot of adrenaline into the bloodstream. This temporarily provides energy—the morning lift so many people get from their first cup of coffee. Adrenaline also dumps stored glycogen (sugar) into the bloodstream, which triggers an outpouring of insulin. This caffeine-triggered rush of sugar and insulin is no help for alcoholics attempting to stabilize their glucose metabolism.

Foods containing refined sugars are also off-limits because they intensify hypoglycemic symptoms (often described as "dry-drunk" behaviors).

Smoking and using snuff or chewing tobacco is bad for everyone, but many alcoholics already have a lower than normal resistance to disease and do not need any more health hazards than they have already accumulated.

Few treatment programs require clients to avoid these substances on the theory that patients should not have to give up anything more than alcohol. It is a sympathetic attitude we don't think our clients can afford.

From the start, our treatment results were dramatic. Even clients who had failed to recover repeatedly in the past did very well. After two years, we knew we were on the right track. Most clients recovered both their sobriety and their health. The time had come to collect scientific data to confirm (or disprove) what we thought was happening. This research became the basis of my Ph.D. dissertation. I collected data on one hundred alcoholic clients chosen at random. Each was followed for up to three and a half years after treatment. Briefly, this is what I found:

- Ninety-eight percent had either an alcoholic parent or close relative. (The other two were adopted, so their genetic heritage was unknown.)
- There were ninety-eight previous treatment experiences among the one hundred patients (some had been treated more than once; others, not at all). Of those previously treated, more than half had relapsed by the third month following their last treatment stay. After one year, only 24 percent had remained sober.
- Of the one hundred clients, eighty-eight had abnormal glucose metabolism (hypoglycemia or diabetes).
- Many were deficient in a number of essential nutrients.
- Seventy-three percent tested positive for allergies to various foods; the most common allergies were to wheat and dairy products.
- Fifty-five percent were sensitive to some environmental chemical,

principally to products containing hydrocarbons, including ethanols and gasoline.

- Twenty-five percent suffered from candida-related complex, a condition stemming from an overcolonization of opportunistic yeast, *Candida albicans,* in the body. CRC can underlie depression, acute fatigue, indigestion, migraine headaches, vaginal and sinus infections, premenstrual syndrome, and impaired immune-system functioning. Alcoholics are particularly susceptible because their high intake of sugar (in the form of alcohol) provides a receptive environment for the growth of these intestinal fungi. Poor nutrition can also set the stage for CRC, as can frequent use of antibiotics to treat the infections to which alcoholics in poor health are prone (antibiotics can upset the natural balance of protective bacteria in the intestinal tract that holds *Candida albicans* in check).

We tabulated symptoms rated by clients as serious to severe upon their entry into the program and again at discharge; mild symptoms were omitted. At entry, a total of 84 percent of the clients reported cravings for alcohol. This figure had dropped to 9 percent by discharge. Table 1 gives a list of the other symptoms at entry and upon discharge.

I wanted to compare the changes in our clients' symptoms to those of clients receiving conventional treatment. Unfortunately, most treatment centers don't publish records on such symptoms. Many of our clients reported that they were not retested for remaining symptoms at discharge from previous treatment programs. However, a 1983 study (D. Mossberg et al.) at St. Goran's Hospital in Stockholm listed symptoms that all patients reported as continuing four to eight weeks after treatment:

- Anxiety
- Insomnia
- Tremors, shakiness
- Dizziness
- Depression
- Impaired cognitive thinking, poor memory

Table 1. Symptoms Reported by HRC Clients

Symptom	Before Treatment	After Treatment
Mood swings	70%	5%
Anxiety, fear	64%	11%
Exhaustion	67%	3%
Irritability	74%	18%
Poor memory	69%	11%
Magnify insignificant events	75%	11%
Reduced initiative	89%	5%
Tremors, shakiness	44%	2%
Dizziness	53%	4%
Depression	61%	5%
Headaches	51%	5%
Insomnia	44%	6%
Chronic fatigue	77%	15%
Cry easily	42%	4%
Physically weak	44%	2%

Here's how our clients compared:

- Eighty-nine percent were free of anxiety by discharge
- Ninety-four percent had no sleep problems
- Ninety-eight percent experienced no tremors or shakiness
- Ninety-six percent were free of dizziness
- Ninety-five percent were depression free

Since our clients and those taking part in the Swedish study all received psychological counseling, it is clear that what made the difference was the Health Recovery Center's biochemical rehabilitation (Figure 3).

My study included two follow-up interviews with each client. The first, at six months, showed that 92 percent were abstinent from

Figure 3. Symptoms Remaining After Treatment: Comparison of Swedish Study with HRC Results

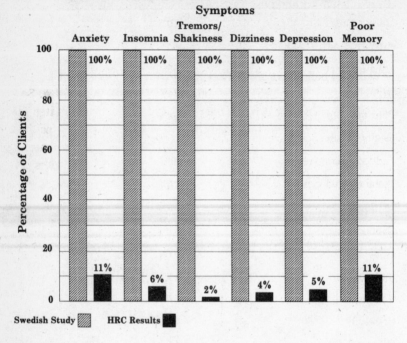

Swedish Study ▨   HRC Results ■

alcohol and that 85 percent had remained continually abstinent since treatment. The second follow-up took place three and a half years after treatment. We located ninety-five of the one hundred clients, and I was thrilled to find that 74 percent remained abstinent. The results of our study were published in the *International Journal of Biosocial and Medical Research*.

At best, conventional treatment results in about 25 percent of clients remaining abstinent at yearly follow-ups. Our success rate has remained about the same as it was when I completed my study: 75 percent, not 25 percent, of our clients recover. They no longer crave alcohol. They are no longer depressed, hyper, or anxious. The memory problems and inability to concentrate that plague so many alcoholics have been banished. Our clients have the energy and self-confidence to handle the challenges of life.

These are the gifts of biochemical repair. I wish this form of treatment were more widely available, but I'm not surprised that it is taking so long. Acceptance of new ideas comes slowly in any field. As Schopenhauer so wisely observed, "All truth passes through three stages. First, it is ridiculed. Second, it is violently opposed. Third, it is accepted as being self-evident."

Although I believe we are fast approaching that third stage, I see no reason why any alcoholic has to suffer needlessly in the interim. So much of the biochemical repair offered at Health Recovery Center is easy to learn. Everything you need to know is contained in the pages to follow, and you can use the book as your personal treatment manual. Your do-it-yourself method may not be as fine-tuned as it would be at the Health Recovery Center, but with the cooperation of your physician, you will come very close.

Your first step will be to determine whether your body chemistry predisposes you to alcoholism and which alcohol biotype fits your symptoms. The results won't be based on your personality or behavior. Your chemistry will tell you all you need to know.

Four

The Difference in Drinkers

Your body holds the key to understanding the effect alcohol has on you. If you have the ability to drink large amounts of alcohol, you have good reason to suspect that you might be predisposed to alcoholism. But, capacity is only part of the story. Alcohol affects brain and body processes in different ways in different people. In this chapter, you'll learn whether or not you are alcoholic and, if so, what kind of alcoholic you are. The following case histories drawn from the files of the Health Recovery Center illustrate three different body chemistries that underlie vulnerability to alcoholism (and one type that may lead to a mistaken diagnosis of alcoholism).

Alan was a party animal in high school and college. Even then he had the capacity to drink heavily without noticeable consequences. In fact, alcohol seemed to stimulate and energize him. Later, in the business world, a few drinks at lunch and dinner served to fuel his professional performance.

Alan was the kind of hard-driving, compulsive person psychologists describe as a Type-A personality: he was ambitious, needed little sleep, and had a strong sex drive. He was proud of his ability to handle alcohol.

For years he wasn't bothered by hangovers and never suspected his supernormal response to alcohol was a red flag signaling trouble down the road. But slowly his body became dependent on alcohol for peak performance. Without it, every cell seemed to feel the letdown. His performance suffered, and he began to crave alcohol.

By the time he was forty-five, he was much less able to withstand the effects of his heavy drinking. He began to experience withdrawal symptoms. Drinking no longer made him feel euphoric or energetic. It simply made him feel normal.

His withdrawal symptoms worsened. He was hyperactive, shaky. His moods and emotions swung wildly from one extreme to another. He blamed his problems on the stress of his job, the inability of his family to understand his needs, and almost every other negative external event he could seize on. His family and colleagues correctly attributed Alan's irritability, mood swings, and the difficulty he had concentrating to his drinking, but they—and he—thought he could and should control it. He began to have blackouts and terrible hangovers, but it was not until he was arrested four times for driving while intoxicated that he admitted that alcohol was destroying him.

Alan's huge capacity for alcohol and the fact that for years it energized him and caused no hangovers indicates that he was born with an alcohol dehydrogenase liver enzyme (II ADH) that enabled his body to metabolize large amounts of alcohol without negative effects. His brain made endorphin-like tetrahydroisoquinolines (THIQs) from alcohol; the THIQs were responsible for both the euphoria he loved and his eventual addiction.

Alan is a II ADH/THIQ alcoholic.

Leonard first drank in high school and remembers how sick alcohol made him until he "learned" to handle it. Unfortunately, that ability was unpredictable. While still in his teens, he totaled the family car

and began accumulating arrests for driving while intoxicated. He
could never predict whether or not a night out would end in another
wild drinking spree. The only thing he could be sure of was that when
he drank heavily, he paid for it the next day with a terrible hangover.
Leonard's father and brothers were affected by alcohol in the same
way, so it didn't occur to him that his drinking pattern was unusual.

When I met Leonard, he had been in Alcoholics Anonymous for
several years and had completed two alcoholic treatment programs.
He had been arrested six times for driving while intoxicated. He was
not yet thirty years old.

Leonard's mother had died a short time earlier. Her death triggered
yet another binge that ended in a bar fight and Leonard's latest arrest
for driving while intoxicated. Leonard sincerely wanted to quit drinking. After his release from jail, he went to his mother's grave and wept,
promising to stay sober, but days later he was drunk again. Now he
was severely depressed, convinced he was a hopeless failure who
would never stay away from alcohol.

His story illustrates the pattern of alcohol allergy/addiction. It takes
about four days for the body to completely rid itself of alcohol. During
this period, withdrawal symptoms in the form of alcohol cravings and
hyperemotional feelings begin to build. Eventually, the victim drinks
to satisfy the cravings and calm his mood. All of these symptoms cease
as soon as he or she reintroduces the addictive substance. When this
type of alcoholic tries to stop drinking, his or her body will seem to
scream for alcohol to banish the withdrawal symptoms. No amount of
counseling, no effort of will can effectively counter the physical and
emotional effects that beset alcoholics like Leonard.

Alcohol-allergic drinkers often become socially disruptive, engaging
in fights and arguments, or become a threat to themselves and others
with dangerous driving, decision-making errors, and even criminal
acts. Alcohol disrupts their normal brain chemistry, causing erratic,
even bizarre behavior. In Leonard's case, this alteration in brain chemistry led to his bar fights and drunken-driving arrests.

The fact that his first drinking experience made him sick was a clear
message that his body couldn't tolerate alcohol. His continued drinking forged a pattern of allergy/addiction: at first, alcohol made him
high as his body reacted to it by producing its own addictive endor-

phins; later, as the alcohol began to leave his system, his body began to crave more to stave off withdrawal symptoms. Both the craving and his emotionality (weeping at his mother's grave, his depression) stemmed from the effect of alcohol withdrawal on his brain.

Leonard is a classic allergic/addicted alcoholic.

Stanley's mother was an alcoholic who also suffered from depression. He was an anxious and depressed child.

Stanley began to drink in his late teens. His first drink was a revelation. For the first time in his life he felt normal and happy. However, his depression returned with more intensity after each drinking episode. He began to drink continually to banish his depression. Finally, he admitted to himself that his drinking was out of control and was ruining his future. His wife finally convinced him to join Alcoholics Anonymous. With sobriety, depression returned. Eventually, Stanley decided that he had a choice between suicide and the bottle. He chose alcohol. Again, his depression miraculously lifted, but soon he found that he had to drink every morning to push depression away.

Once again, he became too ill to function. His career and marriage were floundering when his wife and family arranged for him to be hospitalized for treatment.

I met him after he completed a series of four inpatient treatment programs. Each time he was released, he immediately began drinking again. He had lost hope of finding effective help. He had spent $50,000 for treatment. His therapists had unearthed an incestuous relationship he had had as a teenager to which they attributed both his depression and his drinking. Now Stanley had this painful memory to add to his guilt and shame.

At this time, he was almost fifty years old. His story suggested to me that he was an omega-6 essential fatty acid (EFA) deficient alcoholic. I was right. Within three weeks he was free of depression for the first time without alcohol. He was ecstatic, although he secretly believed it would all collapse shortly. It hasn't.

Sometimes even two or three glasses of wine made Maryanne sick. She became light-headed and uncoordinated and, occasionally, she vomited. Yet her anticipation of that first drink could be overpowering. Her desire for and reaction to alcohol was worse before her menstrual period, a time when she also craved chocolate.

When I met Maryanne, she was afraid she was becoming an alcoholic like her father, a longtime AA member who occasionally falls off the wagon. I didn't think so. Maryanne had a relatively low tolerance for alcohol, a pretty good indication that the problem lies elsewhere.

Maryanne had an inherited predisposition to hypoglycemia (low blood sugar). As a result, her brain does not get a steady supply of its only fuel, glucose (blood sugar). Hypoglycemia is common among alcoholics and can be passed on to their nonalcoholic children (it also occurs in families with no history of alcoholism). Maryanne's craving for chocolates and alcohol was caused by low glucose levels in her brain. Her cravings often occurred when she was premenstrual because hormonal shifts at that time of the month lower blood-sugar levels. Indeed, premenstrual syndrome can stem from an acute hypoglycemic state that develops just before menstruation.

Soon after Maryanne drank the alcohol she craved, she felt a lift, but it didn't last long. Because alcohol is a potent sugar that enters the bloodstream through the stomach wall (it doesn't have to be digested like a candy bar), hypoglycemics feel a fast emotional lift as much-needed glucose surges to their brains.

To maintain this up feeling, hypoglycemics must keep drinking. Otherwise, the insulin produced in response to the glucose infusion will push down blood-sugar levels, resulting in mild insulin shock.

In Maryanne's case, the combined impact of alcohol's toxic effect on her glucose metabolism and sensitive body chemistry can and does make her ill. If this is your problem, you may seem drunk after only one or two drinks.

A glucose tolerance test confirmed what I suspected about Maryanne. She was not alcoholic, but she was severely hypoglycemic. Luckily, this type of alcohol problem is not true alcoholism and lends itself very successfully to treatment.

These case histories describe the four most common categories of drinkers who have sought help at the Health Recovery Center during the past ten years. A new biotype might be identified in the future, but, in all likelihood, if you have a problem with alcohol, you fall into one of the four groups. If there are alcoholics on both sides of your family, you may find that you fit into two categories. If so, the one that predominates, even slightly, is the one to work with as you embark on this program.

The first step will be to test yourself to determine whether or not you are an alcoholic and, if so, what kind you are. Once you know your chemical traits, you can choose the right course to restore your health. Establishing your underlying physical vulnerability has another major advantage: it takes all the shame out of being alcoholic. There is no reason to be embarrassed about the hand your genes have dealt you.

Establishing Your Biotype

The biotype survey below will help you identify your alcohol biotype. You may find that more than one statement applies. Circle any that are true for you *today*.

Biotype Survey

A. *Physiologic Response*

1. Alcohol quickly makes me light-headed, spacey, uncoordinated. It has always affected me this way.
2. Even a little alcohol makes me sick. This has always been true.
3. When drinking, I have lots of energy and perform better.
4. At first, alcohol exhilarates me; then I may lose control and drink until drunk.
5. In the past, alcohol always gave me a lift; now it just takes away my shakiness and makes me feel normal.
6. After only a few drinks, I usually feel sedated by alcohol.
7. I can overcome my depression by drinking alcohol, but afterward the depression seems worse.
8. (Women only) I need and use more alcohol premenstrually.
9. Usually, I can't feel the effect of my first one or two drinks.
10. Now alcohol lifts my depression temporarily. In my earlier drinking years, I did not suffer from depression.

B. *First Experience*

1. I remember the first time I drank alcohol; I liked the feeling it gave me.
2. My first drinking experience was not good; I reacted badly to alcohol.
3. I can't remember my first drinking experience.
4. From my first taste, alcohol has had no appeal for me.

C. *Hangovers*

1. All my drinking years I have usually felt miserable the morning after heavy alcohol use.
2. I rarely have hangovers.
3. I frequently suffer from depression after a night of heavy drinking.
4. I never got hangovers in my early years of heavy drinking, but now I do.
5. I don't get hangovers from my habitual light drinking.
6. I do get uncomfortable even with very little alcohol. This has always been true.

D. *Patterns*

1. I drink six or more eight-ounce glasses of beer a day or the equivalent in wine (six four-ounce glasses) or hard liquor (six drinks, each containing one and one-half ounces of alcohol) and do not get hangovers.
2. I usually can't predict or control how much alcohol I will drink at one time.
3. I may go for days, weeks, or months without alcohol, but when I drink I tend to binge for several days. This has been my usual pattern since I began drinking.
4. I rarely want more than two or three drinks at one time.
5. I do not drink because I dislike the way even a little alcohol affects me.
6. I often experience an urge to drink at the end of the workday following job-related exposure to fumes from gasoline, printer's ink, house paint, hydrocarbons, or formaldehyde.

7. I recognize that I can regularly drink a lot, need little sleep, have a strong sex drive, and tend to be a compulsive Type-A personality.
8. (Women only) I drink quite moderately except before my period, when my need for alcohol seems to increase.
9. I have never been a heavy drinker, but I notice if I haven't eaten, I can get drunk on one or two drinks.
10. I drink daily (or frequently) to avoid depression.

E. Heredity

1. No one on either side of my family has regularly consumed large amounts of alcohol.
2. I have a close maternal and/or paternal relative who drinks (or formerly drank) alcohol in large amounts.
3. I am of Scandinavian, Celtic, Welsh, or Scottish ancestry and have drinking relatives who suffer from depression.
4. I am adopted and do not know my biological parentage.
5. My family may or may not be teetotalers, but my biological origins are predominantly northern European or native American.
6. My family is from a southern Mediterranean country.
7. A close relative is a heavy drinker, but even one or two drinks makes me spacey.
8. I am of Oriental descent. My relatives and I become flushed, dizzy, and nauseated from very little alcohol.

F. Personality Effects

1. My personality and behavior often change markedly when I drink. This effect has been my response to alcohol since I began drinking.
2. My personality and behavior now change markedly when I drink. This was not true in my earlier years of drinking.
3. I mellow out and grow sleepy on a few drinks.
4. I feel revved up and can often party all night when I'm drinking with few or no signs of intoxication.
5. I sometimes get into fights when drinking a lot. This has been true almost from the time I began drinking.

6. I use alcohol to control anxiety whenever possible.
7. I can count on alcohol to lift my lifelong depression temporarily.
8. My behavior sometimes gets bizarre when I drink.
9. I dislike drinking alcohol because it physically upsets me; it does not alter my personality.
10. I feel a quick sense of well-being from my first drink or two but can't handle more than that without feeling spacey and lightheaded.

G. Tolerance

1. I have always had a high tolerance for alcohol and can drink large amounts without problems.
2. I have been able to increase my tolerance for alcohol markedly over time, handling it supernormally with minimal hangovers.
3. I have no ability to handle a lot of alcohol.
4. My tolerance for alcohol has gone down recently. It was much higher for many years.
5. I am inconsistent in how much alcohol I can handle. Often I cannot predict or control how much I will drink.

Your responses in four or five of the seven categories should be consistent within a particular alcohol biotype. If you are over forty and have been drinking heavily for several decades, you may have circled many allergic/addicted responses as well as II ADH/THIQ answers. This would indicate that your drinking has damaged your immune system, your body's defense against disease. However, you are predominantly a II ADH/THIQ alcoholic. In rare cases, a person will be a combination of biotypes if there are different kinds of alcoholics on each side of his or her family.

Scoring

A. Physiologic response

Nonalcoholic chemistry	A6
Nonalcoholic (alcohol-intolerant) chemistry	A2
Nonalcoholic hypoglycemic chemistry	A1, A8
II ADH/THIQ alcoholic chemistry	A3, A5, A9, A10
Allergic/addicted alcoholic chemistry	A4
Omega-6 EFA deficient alcoholic chemistry	A7

B. First experience

Nonalcoholic chemistry	B3
Nonalcoholic (alcohol-intolerant) chemistry	B2, B4
Nonalcoholic hypoglycemic chemistry	B3
II ADH/THIQ alcoholic chemistry	B1
Allergic/addicted alcoholic chemistry	B2
Omega-6 EFA deficient alcoholic chemistry	B1

C. Hangovers

Nonalcoholic chemistry	C5
Nonalcoholic (alcohol-intolerant) chemistry	C6
Nonalcoholic hypoglycemic chemistry	C6
II ADH/THIQ alcoholic chemistry	C2, C4
Allergic/addicted alcoholic chemistry	C1, C3
Omega-6 EFA deficient alcoholic chemistry	C3

D. Patterns

Nonalcoholic chemistry	D4
Nonalcoholic (alcohol-intolerant) chemistry	D5
Nonalcoholic hypoglycemic chemistry	D8, D9
II ADH/THIQ alcoholic chemistry	D1, D7
Allergic/addicted alcoholic chemistry	D2, D3, D6
Omega-6 EFA deficient alcoholic chemistry	D10

Scoring *(Continued)*

E. Heredity

Nonalcoholic chemistry	E1, E6, E8
Nonalcoholic (alcohol-intolerant) chemistry	E8
Nonalcoholic hypoglycemic chemistry	E1, E7
Alcoholic chemistry (possible to probable)	E2, E5
Omega-6 EFA deficient (possible, probable)	E2, E3
Unidentifiable chemistry	E4, E5

F. Personality effects

Nonalcoholic chemistry	F3
Nonalcoholic hypoglycemic chemistry	F3, F10
II ADH/THIQ alcoholic chemistry	F2, F4, F6
Allergic/addicted alcoholic chemistry	F1, F5, F6, F8
Omega-6 EFA deficient alcoholic chemistry	F7

G. Tolerance

Nonalcoholic chemistry	G3
Nonalcoholic (alcohol-intolerant) chemistry	G3
Nonalcoholic hypoglycemic chemistry	G3
II ADH/THIQ or omega-6 EFA deficient	G1, G2, G4
Allergic/addicted alcoholic chemistry	G5

The Characteristics of Your Biotype

1. Nonalcoholic Chemistry (Normal Drinker)

A6 With a few (one to four) drinks, alcohol has a sedating effect on you.

B3 You probably have no outstanding memory of your first alcoholic drink or your reaction to it.

C5 Your alcohol use is usually light; hangovers are rare.

D4 Typically, two to four drinks are enough for you.

E1 Usually, no one on either side of your family drinks or has frequently drunk large amounts of alcohol.

E6 Some of your biological relatives come from southern Mediterranean areas of Europe.

F3 Getting sedated by alcohol is the typical response of a nonalcoholic.

G3 Your ability to "keep up with the boys" when drinking at parties is poor. You would consider it punishment to have to drink twelve beers or a pint of vodka daily and simply couldn't do it, no matter what your personality or character. You are blessed with the chemistry of a nonalcoholic drinker.

2. Nonalcoholic (Alcohol-Intolerant) Chemistry

A2 Drinking even a little alcohol tends to make you dizzy or nauseated or causes flushing or other negative reactions.

B2 Your first drinking experience made you sick.

B4 Because of alcohol's negative effects on you, it has never had any appeal.

C6 Even a little alcohol may give you lingering effects the next day.

D5 Because you dislike the way even a little alcohol affects you, you don't drink.

E8 Your family may be of Oriental extraction and you may possess only one alcohol dehydrogenase enzyme in your liver.

F3 Getting sedated by alcohol is the typical response of a nonalcoholic.

F9 Alcohol offers you no rewarding highs; it only upsets you physically.

G3 You learned quickly that you are alcohol intolerant and you avoid drinking.

3. Nonalcoholic Hypoglycemic Chemistry (May Mistakenly Be Labeled Alcoholic

A1 A little alcohol tends to make you light-headed, spacey, uncoordinated.

A8 If you are a female hypoglycemic you often want and use more alcohol premenstrually; your altered hormonal levels depress glucose metabolism, resulting in severe sugar cravings. Alcohol can temporarily correct this by supplying your brain with glucose, its vital fuel.

B3 Your first drinking experience probably does not stand out in your memory.

C6 You usually get a hangover from moderate drinking because alcohol triggers an outpouring of insulin, which creates mild to severe insulin shock and symptoms of fatigue, confusion, depression, and irritability.

D8 If you are a woman, you may drink more alcohol premenstrually.

D9 The effects of one or two drinks on your empty stomach are dramatic. You almost certainly feel a quick lift followed shortly thereafter by light-headedness, confusion, grogginess, clumsiness, and weakness.

E1 Quite possibly, no one in your family is a heavy drinker. Or . . .

E7 A close relative may be alcoholic, but even a few drinks makes you spacey. In certain alcoholic families, one or two children may inherit the tendency to abnormal glucose metabolism (hypoglycemia) but be spared the high tolerance for alcohol that can lead to alcoholism.

F3 You may be the type of hypoglycemic who tends to become light-headed and sleepy rather quickly as a result of drinking alcohol.

F10 You usually feel a quick sense of well-being from a drink or two.

G3 You never could handle much alcohol. You don't need much to raise blood-sugar levels; a drink or two gives you the temporary lift you seek.

4. II ADH/THIQ Alcoholic Chemistry

A3 Alcohol gives you energy and improves your performance. Or . . .

A5 It used to do this, but now it just stops the shakes and restores you to normal.

A9 You need several drinks to get the feeling you seek.

A10 Alcohol is stimulating the production of endorphins; gradually, this will inhibit natural production of these opiates. Depression can develop as natural endorphins become less available; drinking temporarily relieves your depression.

B1 Your first drinking experiences were pleasant; alcohol didn't make you sick.

C2,C4 Alcohol causes few adverse effects; your hangovers were rare in the heyday of your drinking, but years or even decades later liver damage changed the picture.

D1 You can handle a lot of alcohol. For many years you did not ordinarily have hangovers or experience other alcohol-related consequences.

D7 Besides your ability to handle a lot of alcohol well, you tend to be a Type-A personality, compulsive with a strong sex drive; you require very little sleep to function efficiently.

E2 A close relative has shown a pattern of high alcohol tolerance.

E5 Your ancestors are predominantly northern European or native American.

F2 After years of handling a lot of alcohol supernormally, you are finally showing signs of the damage alcohol is doing to your brain and nervous system.

F4 Alcohol serves to rev up rather than sedate you; you can party for long periods with few or no signs of intoxication.

F6 Alcohol helps you handle situations that make you anxious.

G1 You had a high tolerance for alcohol even as a teenager. Or . . .

G2 Your tolerance increased markedly with continual use of alcohol. Or . . .

G4 Your high tolerance of yesteryear has declined after a long drinking career.

5. Allergic/Addicted Alcoholic Chemistry

A4 Alcohol will exhilarate you at first, but you often lose control and may drink until drunk.

B2 You probably can remember getting sick after your first drinking experience. At the time, your body was able to tell you how it felt about alcohol. With repeated use, your body was forced to adapt and accommodate alcohol. The result is the altered response of allergy/addiction.

C1 You usually have serious aftereffects the morning following heavy drinking because of the toxicity of alcohol to your allergic body.

C3 depression usually follows a night of heavy drinking.

D2 You often can't predict or control how much you will drink at one time because alcohol quickly alters your brain's ability to make choices.

D3 You may go without alcohol for days, weeks, or even months, but when you drink, you tend to binge, sometimes for several days.

D6 Daily exposure to such chemicals as gasoline, formaldehyde, printer's ink, and hydrocarbons can easily intoxicate your sensitive brain and set off cravings for alcohol. If you work around these chemicals you may notice an overwhelming urge to drink immediately after work.

E2 Typically, you have a close relative with a similar drinking pattern. Or . . .

E5 Your relatives are all teetotalers—for good reason. Chances are you are of predominantly northern European or native American background.

F1 Your personality and behavior are often dramatically affected by alcohol because your brain and nervous system are easily disrupted by alcohol's toxicity.

F5 When drinking, you often engage in arguments and bar fights with anyone, even total strangers.

F6 Alcohol tends to mediate your high levels of anxiety and is your preferred way to deal with stress.

F8 The physical changes alcohol triggers in your allergic brain can result in irrational or bizarre behavior; contrary to appearances, you have little control over these actions once you are locked into this altered brain state.

G5 You often can't control how much you drink.

6. Omega-6 EFA (Essential Fatty Acid) Deficient Chemistry

A7 You know you can temporarily relieve depression by drinking alcohol.

B1 Your first drinking experience produced immediate relief from long-standing depression.

C3 Your depression returns after you stop drinking.

D10 You drink daily (or frequently) to prevent depression from returning.

E2 You have relatives who are alcoholics and/or depressed; there may have been some suicides in your family.

E3 Your ancestry is predominantly Scandinavian, Irish, Welsh, or Scottish.

F7 You have come to depend on alcohol for relief from depression present since childhood.

G1 Your tolerance for alcohol probably has increased over the years. Or . . .

G4 Your tolerance may be much reduced after years of drinking, which has caused liver damage.

What's Next?

If you clearly fall into an alcoholic category, you now have the opportunity to rewrite your future. You may decide to keep drinking even though your alcohol biotype indicates that you are headed for disaster. I hope not. You are vulnerable to alcohol and will become addicted in the future if you aren't already. True physical addiction cannot be managed into social drinking.

Since alcoholism is progressive, your drinking habits won't improve; they won't even stay the same. *They will get worse.* Your physical need for alcohol will gradually speak so loud that no act of will can overcome it. Life will become an unending quest for the normalizing lift alcohol provides, even though it will be destroying your health and sanity. Please remember that most alcoholics today *do not* recover. They die prematurely from alcohol-induced diseases.

In the chapters to come, you will learn how to break this addiction and end your cravings once and for all. You will learn how to repair the harm alcohol has done to your brain and body. Without repair, the damage will continue for months and even years after you stop drinking. All too often, this emotional and physical misery leads alcoholics back to the bottle in the quest for relief. You hold in your hands the tools to help you repair this damage now. These techniques have been used successfully at Health Recovery Center for the past ten years. They have helped many others. They may save your life.

Five

Week One:
Assessing the Damage

You are about to embark on a seven-week program that will change your life. I have seen it happen over and over again among the hundreds of alcoholics we treat at Health Recovery Center every year. I'm sure they, like you, had some doubts about whether this program really was the solution to their problems. You will soon see for yourself that it succeeds beyond your dreams.

You will find that it is possible to stop drinking without battling overwhelming cravings for alcohol. For the first time, your body won't be at war with your mind, screaming for a drink and undermining your willpower. You should start to feel better even while you are in the midst of detoxification, when you'll be taking a variety of nutritional supplements to begin your biological repair and quench any cravings for alcohol.

Your physical recovery will accelerate after detox as you begin the full-fledged repair program. You will still be taking a lot of nutritional supplements—the amount depends on your assessment of your particular needs. You will also be changing your diet to control the hypoglycemia that so often underlies alcoholism. You should begin to reap the rewards of this healthy new life-style almost immediately. Your mental and physical functioning will improve swiftly and steadily as your repair program progresses.

Everyone needs the basic repair program and the diet. In addition, there are sixteen nutrient formulas designed to help you overcome specific problems. You may need some, all, or none of these formulas.

I know you'll be tempted to leaf through the pages ahead and zero in on those parts that intrigue you most, but it's very important for you to follow the program in the order in which it is presented. Read through the book carefully before you decide what you need and what you don't.

Before you begin, please ask your mate, a relative, or a good friend to help you. I can't stress enough how important it is—and how much easier it will make things for you—to have someone at your side to guide and support you through the weeks ahead. With this in mind, I would like to address a few words to your companion on this journey.

"This Time It Will Be Different"

If you've heard those words before, you may be skeptical about this time, too. But take *my* word for it: this time it really will be different. This program is unlike any treatment your spouse, friend, lover, or relative has tried before. For the first time, treatment will break through the physical addiction to alcohol to bring your loved one to a new and comfortable state of well-being. You can help enormously by stressing to him or her the physical regeneration in store and the importance of biological repair to mental and physical health.

This is not a time for recriminations. It is not a time to dwell on the mistakes and failures brought on by alcoholism. You may have been advised to separate yourself from the alcoholic's problems and struggles, to let him or her find the way when ready. Other diseases do not drive loved ones away, but all too often alcoholics too ill to help themselves are abandoned by family and friends unable or unwilling to cope with what they erroneously believe is a condition that can be controlled by willpower or self-discipline. If you have read the preceding chapters, you now recognize the true nature of alcoholism. You know you're dealing with someone who is physically sick. Now you have the answers you have sought or prayed for in the past. This program works, and it will work better with your help.

Read through the program and help guide your "patient" through its various stages. Your role is to offer encouragement and emphasize the payoff to come—renewed health, energy, and mental stability. Before you know it, you'll find that the person you love is back with you in body, mind, and spirit, free from alcoholism's numbing and deadly grasp.

Getting Started on Your Recovery

In order to personalize your recovery plan, you must first assess your health. You will learn a lot about where you stand by completing the questionnaires that begin on page 66. But your first step is to make an appointment with your doctor for some medical tests that will reveal any damage alcohol has inflicted on your body. You should have the following tests:

- Complete blood count
- Chemistry profile
- Thyroid function
- Urinalysis
- Five-hour glucose tolerance test
- Serum zinc and copper levels
- Candida-antibody assay
- Serum histamine
- Food allergy assay
- Hair analysis
- Amino-acid analysis

Don't let this long list scare you. Most of the tests require no more than a sample of your blood. Only one, the glucose tolerance test, is time-consuming—you will have to spend part of a day at the doctor's office or lab. At the end of this chapter you'll find a complete description of each of these tests and what they entail.

If you can't have the tests done at this time, you can still follow the program. In fact, I urge you to begin it, tests or no tests. Laboratory results can help fine-tune repair, but it is more important to treat your alcoholism now than to put it off until you can assemble all the relevant medical data.

Choosing a Doctor

As you go about scheduling your tests, you may discover that not all doctors think alike about the importance of hypoglycemia, allergies, food sensitivities/intolerances, candida-related complex, and certain thyroid abnormalities. There are two distinct camps in the field of allergy—represented by the American Academy of Allergy and Immunology and the American College of Allergists—each with different opinions on the importance of food allergies and value of food-allergy testing. There are also physicians who specialize in clinical ecology, the diagnosis and treatment of sensitivities to chemicals and environmental pollutants as well as food allergies. These doctors are particularly attuned to the problems of allergic/addicted alcoholics. Don't make too much of these differing medical views; there is no right or wrong here.

If your family doctor does not routinely test for food allergies or candida-related complex, does not use hair analysis to identify mineral deficiencies or an excess of toxic metals in the body, or is not familiar with research linking alcoholism and hypoglycemia, you can get a referral to a physician who is knowledgeable in these areas by contacting one of the following medical organizations:

The American College for the Advancement in Medicine
23121 Verdugo Drive, Suite 204
Laguna Hills, CA 92543
(714) 583-7666

The American Holistic Medical Association
4101 Lake Boone Terrace, Suite 201
Raleigh, NC 27607
(919) 787-5146

The American Academy of Environmental Medicine
P.O. Box 16106
Denver, CO 80216
(303) 622-9755

Schedule your appointment as soon as possible; within the next week would be ideal. If you can't see a doctor at this time, don't give up. This program will still work for you, although it won't be as finely tuned as it would if you had the test results to work with to personalize repair.

Getting a Fix on Alcoholism

Once you have scheduled your medical tests, set aside some time to complete the questionnaires in Charts 1 to 3. If you are completely honest, your replies will give you a new perspective on your alcoholism. You will see, perhaps for the first time, where it came from and what it has done to you emotionally and physically. Each test page is followed by an explanation of the questions being asked. The comments and examples reflect what I would tell you if you were sitting here in my office about to take the tests.

Chart 1: History of Alcohol Use

Be objective as you chart the patterns and consequences of your alcohol use in the spaces provided on Chart 1. Describe events as facts, not personal failures. Use more paper if you need it.

Alcohol / Drugs Used

In the first category, list any addictive drugs you have taken or are taking now. Check the list below. If you have *ever* used any of the drugs mentioned, be sure to write them in the appropriate space.

1. Alcohol (beer, wine, liquor)
2. Marijuana/hashish

Chart 1. History of Alcohol Use

Age	Alcohol/ Drugs Used	Typical Amounts Used	Frequency of Use	Consequences of Use	Physical Emotional Spiritual	Financial Occupational Legal
Teens: 10–20						
Young Adult: 20–30						
"Prime Time" Adult: 30–40						
Middle-Age Adult: 40–55						
Senior Adult: 55 and Above						

3. Barbiturates (sleeping pills), including Seconal, Nembutal, Amytal, Butisol
4. Chloral hydrates, including Somnos
5. Hypnotics, including Dalmane, Doriden, Quaalude
6. Tranquilizers such as Ativan, Valium, Librium, Xanax, Tranxene, Serax, Centrax, Paxipam
7. Stimulants such as Benzedrine, Didrex, Dexedrine, Dexamyl, Tenuate, Ritalin, Preludin, Dexatrim, Prolamine
8. Cocaine, crack
9. Opiates (painkillers), including codeine, Demerol, Percodan, Nubain, Darvon, Talwin, morphine, Dilaudid
10. Heroin
11. Hallucinogens, including LSD, PCP, mescaline
12. Inhalants such as glue, paint thinner
13. Nicotine (cigarettes, chewing tobacco, cigars, pipes)
14. Caffeine, including coffee, tea, colas, chocolate

If any of these drugs was prescribed, note whether you renewed your prescription or sought additional prescriptions from a second doctor beyond the original intent and need.

People with addictive chemistries often use drugs other than alcohol. This is particularly true of younger people. Most professionals who treat drug abuse recognize that it isn't a sign of a flawed character or psychological weakness. More likely, it suggests that you were seeking better living through chemistry. Your physical vulnerability to alcohol addiction can also trap you into abusing other drugs. As you know, the longer you use an addictive drug, the less of a lift you get. Over time, your body demands more and more to feel normal. This physical entrapment can lead to addiction to either alcohol or another chemical substance.

In describing your history, note the kinds of drugs you like best. This will give you a clue to what you are trying to alter in your own chemistry. For example, we know that teenage marijuana users tend to be restless and hyperactive. Marijuana mellows them out. Amphetamine users may have little natural energy or stamina; the drugs stimulate production of steroids that create the illusion of unlimited natural pep. Heroin users claim that the drug reduces their anxiety and helps them feel normal.

Most alcoholics are drawn to minor tranquilizers like Valium, Librium, and Ativan because these drugs have effects similar to alcohol. You may have noticed that combining alcohol with any of these tranquilizers is like having two or three drinks for every one poured, an effect called "cross-tolerance." In the 1970s, many abstinent AA members took Valium prescribed by their doctors to help them stay sober. But they found that Valium withdrawal takes a month or two, during which they were prey to free-floating anxiety, insomnia, depression, and nervousness. Most doctors now know better than to prescribe minor tranquilizers like Valium for alcoholics except temporarily, during detoxification.

Typical Amounts Used

Note whether you drink beer, wine, or hard liquor and how many drinks you have per day: one to three, four to six, seven to twelve, or more than twelve.

Frequency of Use

Describe your current (during the last six months) frequency of use of alcohol in the following terms: less than once a month, one to three times monthly, weekly, several days a week, or daily.

Then note your longest period of abstinence in the past six months and indicate how many days out of the last month you used alcohol.

Consequences of Use

This section of your history is very important. If you are honest with yourself, you'll begin to see the connection between your alcohol abuse and the way the events of your life unfolded.

Physical consequences can include

- Continual cravings
- Insomnia
- High blood pressure
- Liver disease
- Diabetes
- Ongoing fatigue

- Nervous exhaustion
- Serious weight gain or loss
- Nervous stomach, ulcers
- Tremors
- Heart palpitations
- Poor memory
- Impaired immune function

Emotional consequences can include

- Depression
- Anxiety
- Confusion
- Chronic worrying
- Mood swings
- Fearfulness
- Irritability
- Paranoia

Spiritual consequences can include

- Lack of feeling centered
- Loss of family ties
- Loss of close friendships
- Loss of spiritual beliefs
- Loss of ties to your church

Financial consequences can include

- Heavy debts
- Inability to save money
- No bank account
- Rejection of loan or credit card applications
- Poor money management
- Inability to provide basic family needs

Occupational consequences can include

- Not working at the level of your training and ability
- Poor work performance
- Missing work or being late

- Being fired from your job
- Inability to keep jobs

Legal consequences can include

- Arrests and/or convictions for driving under the influence of alcohol
- Marital separation and/or divorce
- Small claims court suits for nonpayment of bills
- Arrest and conviction for passing bad checks
- Arrest and conviction for fraud
- Arrest and conviction for shoplifting or other thefts

Be sure to answer the same questions for each of the five age categories. Be honest as you complete the questionnaire. You are the only one who will see your answers. Your history will help you see how profoundly alcohol has influenced your life and the effect it has had on your potential and ability to attain your professional and personal goals.

Chart 2: Genetic History

Completing the genetic-history questionnaire in Chart 2 can be a revelation. It will show you where your alcoholism came from and will help you see which lab tests may be particularly enlightening.

Use the chart to track your heredity. Record your paternal history on the left side and maternal history on the right. Do not include relatives by marriage who are not biologically related to you.

Nationality

Your nationality is important because certain ethnic groups are particularly vulnerable to alcoholism. You may be surprised to learn that there is a direct relationship between the rate of alcoholism among an ethnic group and the length of time that group has been exposed to alcohol. People from the Mediterranean areas of Europe have been drinking alcohol for more than seven thousand years. Today, they have a very low (10 percent) susceptibility to alcoholism. Those from

Chart 2. Genetic History

	Paternal	Maternal	Siblings
Nationality:			
Alcoholism:			
Drug dependency:			
Depression:			
Diabetes:			
Mental illness:			
Allergies:			
Obesity/ eating disorders:			

northern European countries, including Ireland, Scotland, Wales, northern parts of Russia and Poland, and the Scandinavian countries, have been using alcohol for only fifteen hundred years. As a result, their susceptibility to alcoholism is measurably higher (between 20 and 40 percent). Native Americans (including Eskimos) had no access to alcohol until three hundred years ago. Their vulnerability to alcoholism is extraordinarily high (between 80 and 90 percent).

The scientific principle of survival of the fittest is at work here. Over many generations, those most susceptible to alcohol have been eliminated. The survivors continue to pass along their low susceptibility. The only deterrent to this process of natural selection is the interbreeding of people from different regions.

Alcoholism

To make an educated guess about some of the drinkers in your family, use this simple criteria: does he or she have an unusually high tolerance for alcohol? Anyone who has never been able to handle much alcohol is not an alcoholic. Those who can and do put away a lot of alcoholic drinks are most likely to have problematic chemistries.

Drug Dependency

Before you decide that you have no family history of drug dependency, think about the Valium Aunt Mary lives on and the painkillers Uncle Joe takes for his chronic aches and pains.

Depression

This condition may be present on either side of your family whether or not it has been formally diagnosed and treated. Record any attempted or accomplished suicides in this category.

Diabetes

This disorder is often seen in a grandparent within an alcoholic family. Native Americans are particularly vulnerable to adult-onset diabetes early in their drinking careers. A glucose tolerance test to identify irregular glucose metabolism is particularly important for anyone with a family history of diabetes.

Mental Illness

Do you have any relatives who suffer(ed) from schizophrenia, nervous breakdowns, or paranoia?

Allergies

Most alcoholics have some family history of allergy. Pollen, dust, mold, and grasses are common offenders. Classic allergic reactions include hives, wheezing, and sneezing. Many people who have an allergic/addicted response to alcohol react adversely to a number of foods, including those containing refined sugars and the grains from which alcohol is made. Becoming overweight is often a sign of food allergy/addiction.

Obesity/Eating Disorders

Bulemia and/or anorexia are often the outcome of years of wrestling with cravings. Young women are most apt to become bulemic in a misguided attempt at weight control, but at any age binge eating can be a sign of food allergy/addiction.

Alcohol/Chemical Dependency Among Siblings

How many of your brothers and sisters are vulnerable to alcoholism? Some may have stopped drinking heavily, but count them as having alcoholic chemistries. Include any siblings who have been addicted to other drugs.

Chart 3: The HRC Symptometer

The self-test in Chart 3 was developed at Health Recovery Center to help us identify our clients' most urgent needs. Be sure to read the following section clarifying the symptoms before beginning the test.

Chart 3. The HRC Symptometer
Week One

	Frequency			
Symptom	**Never 0**	**Mild 1**	**Moderate 2**	**Severe 3**
1. Cravings for alcohol	___	___	___	___
2. Uses alcohol regularly	___	___	___	___
3. Tendency to allergies, asthma, hay fever, rashes	___	___	___	___
4. Bad dreams	___	___	___	___
5. No dream recall	___	___	___	___
6. Unstable moods, frequent mood swings	___	___	___	___
7. Blurred vision	___	___	___	___
8. Frequent thirst	___	___	___	___
9. Bruises easily	___	___	___	___
10. Confusion	___	___	___	___
11. Nervous stomach	___	___	___	___
12. Poor sleep, insomnia, waking up during the night	___	___	___	___
13. Nervous exhaustion	___	___	___	___
14. Indecision	___	___	___	___
15. Can't work under pressure	___	___	___	___
16. Cravings for sweets	___	___	___	___
17. Depression	___	___	___	___
18. Feelings of suspicion, paranoia	___	___	___	___
19. Light-headedness, dizziness	___	___	___	___
20. Anxiety	___	___	___	___
21. Fearfulness	___	___	___	___
22. Tremors, shakes	___	___	___	___

Chart 3. The HRC Symptometer
Week One (Continued)

Symptom	Frequency			
	Never 0	Mild 1	Moderate 2	Severe 3
23. Night sweats	___	___	___	___
24. Heart palpitations	___	___	___	___
25. Compulsive, obsessive, driven	___	___	___	___
26. Manic-depressive (cyclical mood changes)	___	___	___	___
27. Suicidal thoughts	___	___	___	___
28. Irritability, sudden anger	___	___	___	___
29. Lack of energy	___	___	___	___
30. Magnifies insignificant events	___	___	___	___
31. Poor memory	___	___	___	___
32. Inability to concentrate	___	___	___	___
33. Sleepy after meals or late in the afternoon	___	___	___	___
34. Chronic worrier.	___	___	___	___
35. Difficulty awakening in the morning	___	___	___	___
Column Totals	___	___	___	___
Test Total	___	___	___	___

INSTRUCTIONS: Check off each symptom in one of the columns to indicate the degree of severity that applies to you. Zero means never, one means mild, two means moderate, and three means severe. Add up the number of checks in each column and multiply by the number printed at the top of each column. Total score equals the sum of all columns. (Scores over 35 are significant.)

Symptometer Checklist

Some of the items on the symptometer checklist are self-explanatory, but most need some clarification:

1. *Cravings for alcohol:* Heavy daily drinkers may say "absolutely none." Of course you don't crave alcohol when you are drinking. But what happens when you go on the wagon?

2, 3, and 4. Self-explanatory.

5. *No dream recall:* This is a sign of inadequate vitamin B_6 (pyridoxine) availability.

6. *Unstable moods, frequent mood swings:* Frequent changes in mood are a symptom of hypoglycemia. As brain levels of glucose fluctuate, so do moods. The changes occur in the course of twenty-four hours, in contrast to the mood swings of manic depression, which occur over weeks or months.

7 and 8. *Blurred vision and frequent thirst:* These symptoms suggest diabetes; a five-hour glucose tolerance test is in order.

9. *Bruises easily:* Frequent black-and-blue marks indicate a deficiency of Vitamin C and bioflavonoids.

10. *Confusion:* Difficulty thinking clearly; HRC clients have described these feelings as "thinking through peanut butter."

11. *Nervous stomach:* Heavy caffeine users and chronic alcohol drinkers often complain of this problem.

12. *Poor sleep:* Difficulty falling asleep (insomnia); waking often during the night; not being able to fall asleep again easily.

13. *Nervous exhaustion:* This means feeling as if you are coming apart at the seams or are strung out emotionally.

14. *Indecision:* Not being able to make up your mind about everyday matters.

15. Self-explanatory.

16. *Craves sweets:* If you are a daily drinker, you probably get all the sugar you want from alcohol. Craving for sweets can occur when you give up alcohol, your main supply of sugar. Bear in mind that nondiet carbonated beverages often contain up to ten teaspoons of sugar; if you're drinking a lot of these sodas, you may be satisfying an unrecognized craving for sweets.

17. *Depression:* This problem sometimes goes unrecognized, espe-

cially in male alcoholics. Measure depression by asking yourself if, when you take your emotional temperature, it often feels sad inside.

18. *Feelings of suspicion, paranoia:* Alcoholics often experience these feelings as a result of altered brain chemistry.

19. *Light-headedness, dizziness:* These are symptoms of hypoglycemia; you may have noticed them in the late mornings or afternoons when your blood sugar drifts too low. Some hypoglycemics also have abnormally low blood pressure and may feel light-headed when they stand up suddenly.

20. *Anxiety:* In this context, anxiety refers to an ongoing state, rather than concern about specific events. Sometimes anxiety precedes alcoholism and is the reason a person seeks relief by drinking.

21. *Fearfulness:* Fear of people and places can be a lifelong condition rooted in the biochemical status of the brain. Alcohol offers temporary relief.

22. *Tremors, shakes:* This means involuntary shaking relieved by alcohol.

23. Self-explanatory.

24. *Heart palpitations:* This can occur among chronic drinkers withdrawing from alcohol.

25. *Compulsive, obsessive, driven:* Are you a Type-A driven personality? Your lab test may show high blood levels of histamine, a brain chemical associated with this type of behavior. Bringing histamine levels back to normal will help. You will learn how in Chapter 9.

26. *Manic-depressive (cyclical mood changes):* A pattern alternating between unnatural exhilaration for weeks and months with severe depression for another period of weeks or months. This cycle is sometimes seen among II ADH/THIQ alcoholics. If you are affected, you should be under a doctor's care. You may need treatment with lithium, a natural element available by prescription.

27. *Suicidal thoughts:* If you rate this symptom high, tell your doctor and a close friend or relative. You will find the help you need to lift your underlying biochemical depression in Chapter 10.

28. *Irritability, sudden anger:* These symptoms also have biochemical roots and a biochemical cure.

29. *Lack of energy:* This is a common symptom of hypoglycemia. Chapters 7 and 8 will give you the tools to eliminate this problem.

30. *Magnifies insignificant events:* Do you blow things out of proportion? Alcoholics often have this tendency as a result of the effect of nutritional deficiencies on the brain.

31. *Poor memory:* By this I mean short-term memory. Do you forget why you came looking for something? Do you continually have to write down appointments and make other notes to yourself? Heavy alcohol use destroys the availability of acetylcholine, a brain chemical essential for memory function, as well as vitamin B_1 (thiamine), a key nutrient for memory recall.

32. *Unable to concentrate:* Do you have trouble reading a book or sticking to a project?

33. *Sleepy after meals:* This is a symptom of food allergy. A meal should give you a lift, not make you sleepy. Sleepiness in the late afternoon may also be caused by declining glucose levels (hypoglycemia).

34. Self-explanatory.

35. *Difficulty awakening in the morning:* This problem occurs among nutritionally malnourished alcoholics. It may also be a symptom of low thyroid function.

Instructions for scoring your symptometer appear at the bottom of Chart 3. Don't feel discouraged if your score is high; it is only a barometer of your emotional and physical state. Once your specific problems are identified, you can get on with the job of repairing the damage. When you have completed your course to recovery, you'll fill out another symptometer. Almost all of the clients at the Health Recovery Center return to the normal range (a score of less than 35) by the time they have completed their recovery program.

Chart 4:
Laboratory Test Request

Before you see your doctor, you should know something about the lab tests you will be having and what they can tell you about your health. We recommend the following tests:

Complete Blood Count

Type: Blood test.

Purpose: To determine if you are anemic, have any acute or chronic infections or blood disorders.

Where available: Most health-care facilities—doctors' offices, clinics, hospitals, and clinical laboratories.

Preparation required: None.

Results: Usually available within a week.

Chemistry Profile

Type: Blood test.

Purpose: To measure blood glucose, total cholesterol, high-density lipoproteins (HDL), low-density lipoproteins (LDL), and triglycerides. The test also yields some information about liver function, indicating whether you may have cirrhosis of the liver or other liver disorders or damage.

Where available: Most health-care facilities.

Preparation required: Do not eat after ten o'clock the night before.

Results: Usually available within one week.

Thyroid Function

Type: Blood test.

Purpose: To assess thyroid function. Low thyroid function is very common among alcoholics. Symptoms include fatigue, slow thinking, depression, hoarseness, dry and flaking skin, cold hands and feet, coarse or brittle hair, fingernails that are ridged and break easily, and sexual problems.

Where available: Most health-care facilities, but see note below.

Chart 4. Laboratory Test Request

_____ Complete blood count

_____ T$_3$, T$_4$, TSH

_____ Five-hour glucose tolerance test

_____ Serum copper

_____ Serum histamine

_____ Hair Analysis**

_____ Amino-acid analysis: neuropsychiatric panel‡

_____ Chemistry profile

_____ Urinalysis

_____ Serum zinc

_____ Candida-antibody assay*

_____ IgG RAST and FICA†

Requested by: _____ M.D.

_____

Address

*ImmunoDiagnostic Laboratories, P.O. Box 5755, San Leandro, CA 94577, (800) 888-1113 or (415) 635-4555.
†Immuno-Nutritional Clinical Laboratories, 7404 Fulton Avenue, North Hollywood, CA 91605-4114, (800) 344-4646 or (818) 780-4720 (in California).
**Omegatech, P.O. Box 44, Troutdale, VA 24378, (800) 437-8888 or (702) 677-3631.
‡Tyson and Associates, 12832 Chadron Avenue, Hawthorne, CA 90250, (800) 433-9750 (in California), (800) 367-7744.

Preparation required: None.

Results: Usually available within one week.

Note: The standard tests of thyroid function measure two components of thyroid hormone: triiodothyronine (T_3) and total thyroxine (T_4). A test for thyroid stimulating hormone (TSH) done on the same blood sample helps determine if thyroid function is normal. In some cases at HRC where these test results have been within normal limits, a new test, the fluorescence activated microsphere assay (FAMA) has revealed the presence of antibodies formed against the thyroid. The FAMA test can also identify changes that precede full-blown hypothyroidism by seven or eight years. The test is available from ImmunoDiagnostic Laboratories in San Leandro, California. Results are usually available within two weeks.

Urinalysis

Type: Urine test.

Purpose: To diagnose diabetes, chronic urinary infections, and kidney problems. Extra sugar in the urine would suggest diabetes; excess white cells indicate urinary infection. The presence of protein or albumen in the sample is a sign of a kidney disorder.

Where available: Most health-care facilities.

Preparation required: None.

Results: Usually available within a week.

Five-Hour Glucose Tolerance Test

Type: Blood and urine. You provide blood and urine samples when you arrive, then you drink a solution of glucose. The blood and urine tests are repeated thirty minutes later and then every hour thereafter for five hours.

Purpose: To detect abnormal glucose metabolism that underlies hypoglycemia or diabetes.

Where available: Most health-care facilities.

Preparation required:

1. Do not drink alcohol or use drugs for at least one week prior to the test.

2. Avoid taking nutritional supplements for forty-eight hours prior to the test.

3. Do not eat or drink anything (except water) after ten o'clock the night before the test. Take no medications. However, if you are under a doctor's care and are taking drugs prescribed for a specific condition, do not stop taking your medication before discussing it with your physician. Do not chew gum. It is very important to maintain this fast before and during the five hours of the test.

4. Cigarettes are cured with three different kinds of sugar. For this reason, smoking will invalidate test results, so don't smoke before or during the test.

5. Take a copy of Chart 5, Hypoglycemia Test Symptoms, to keep a written record of any symptoms that occur during the test. Note the time you experience them. Symptoms that continue after the test ends and you have eaten a meal suggest a cerebral allergy reaction to sugar and/or the corn from which the sugar was made.

6. When the test is over, eat some fruit or drink some orange juice to restore your blood-sugar levels before you start for home.

Results: Usually available within a week.

Note: Your glucose tolerance test can be a surprising experience. You may react in ways you didn't anticipate. The three case histories below will give you an idea of the type of reactions that can occur.

Case 1:

Jim felt dazed and hungry when his glucose tolerance test ended. As instructed, he had brought a banana and a package of walnuts to eat before he left the lab, but he couldn't remember why he was carrying the brown paper bag. Out in the street, he was overtaken by panic. He couldn't remember where he was or where he wanted to go. Reading the familiar names on the street signs didn't help. After a terrifying few minutes, he looked inside the lunch bag. He bolted down the banana, and his memory began to return. Jim's problem is not unusual: glucose levels in his brain had dropped so low that he became totally but temporarily confused.

Chart 5. Hypoglycemia Test Symptoms

	Fasting	½ Hour	1 Hour	2 Hour	3 Hour	4 Hour	5 Hour	6 Hour
Gasping for air								
Headachy								
Tired								
Shaky								
Irritable								
Anxious								
Weak								
Paranoid								
Depressed								
Nervous								
Sweating								
Digestive disturbances								
Worrying								
Clumsy								
Lack of concentration								
Suicidal thoughts								
Exhausted								
Heart palpitations								
Forgetful								

Chart 5. Hypoglycemia Test Symptoms (*Continued*)

	Fasting	½ Hour	1 Hour	2 Hour	3 Hour	4 Hour	5 Hour	6 Hour
Ears ringing								
Restless								
Light-headed								
Indecisive								
Cold hands/feet								
Blurred vision								
Joint pain								
Loss of appetite								
Sugar cravings								
Alcohol cravings								
Food cravings								
Other								

Developed by Janet Dahlem—Health Matters, Inc.

Case 2:

During the first hours of his test, Mark watched cartoons on television with other patients in the lab's waiting room. He began to feel increasingly irritated with the program and the patients who were watching it. But when someone got up and changed the channel, he jumped up shouting obscenities. Later, he said that his rage made no sense to him, but he hadn't been able to control it. He compared his reaction to his outbursts at his wife, when he would suddenly start arguing over nothing. In Mark's case, adrenaline released to counter low brain levels of glucose triggered the body's fight or flight response to stress. His brain, low on glucose, was not capable of the rational thought needed to control his outburst.

Case 3:

Three hours into Jane's test, she was overcome by depression and began to sob. The faces of the other patients seemed distorted and objects began to change shape before her eyes. The lab technician halted the test and persuaded Jane to drink some orange juice and eat the food she had brought.

Although she felt better after eating, Jane's sadness and emotional instability lingered all day. These long-lasting symptoms indicate a cerebral allergic response to the glucose. I'll tell you all about this condition in Chapter 11.

Note: A number of medications or disorders, listed below, affect blood glucose levels. Be sure to tell the doctor if any apply to you. (For accuracy and with the assumption that you will recognize the name of a drug you take or disorder you suffer from, I am using the medical terminology.) The following drugs and disorders can *increase* blood glucose levels:

Chlorpromazine, diuretics, epinephrine, indomethacin, marijuana, nicotinic acid, ACTH, adrenal steroids, androgens, estrogens (including birth-control pills), glucagon, growth hormone, thyroid medication (such as thyroxine), coffee, smoking.

Emotional stress, infection, pregnancy, aldosteronism, anacidity, arthritis, gastrectomy, hypertension, jejunectomy, liver disease, kidney inflammation (nephritis), obesity, pheochromocytoma, prolonged inactivity.

The following drugs and disorders can *decrease* blood glucose levels:

Alcohol, aspirin, barbiturates, bishydroxycoumarin, chloramphenicol, Librium, MAO inhibitors, oxyphenbutazone, phenylbutazone, Valium.

Fever, islet-cell tumors of the pancreas, Addison's disease, strenuous physical exercise.

Serum Zinc and Copper Levels

Type: Blood test.
Purpose: To diagnose a deficiency of zinc or toxic levels of copper.

Alcohol destroys zinc. Chronic alcohol consumption and high sugar intake often force the body to excrete zinc, which can lead to a deficiency. Inadequate zinc levels can cause an increase in copper levels, which in turn may result in "psychological" disorders, including paranoia.

If you have been taking oral contraceptives or other drugs containing estrogen, expect to see your zinc levels drop below normal. Without adequate zinc, wounds heal slowly and the ability to taste and smell diminishes. Diabetics and hypoglycemics often complain of cold hands and feet, caused by both poor circulation and low levels of zinc. White marks on your fingernails and stretch marks on your hips, thighs, breasts, or abdomen are signs of zinc deficiency.

Where Available: Most health-care facilities.

Preparation required: None.

Results: Usually available within one week.

Candida-Antibody Assay

Type: Blood test.

Purpose: To detect candida-related complex (CRC) by measuring levels of three different antibodies: IgG, IgA, and IgM. Normally, these levels are 100 MONA (measure of normal activity) units or below. In patients with CRC, one or more of the antibody counts can rise to 200 units or higher.

Where available: Your doctor can draw the blood sample and send it for analysis to the lab we use, ImmunoDiagnostic Laboratories.

Preparation required: None.

Results: Usually available in two weeks.

Serum Histamine Testing

Type: Blood test.

Purpose: To measure levels of histamine, an important body chemical involved in allergic reactions: Inside the brain, histamine is a regulator of important neurotransmitters.

Where available: Most medical laboratories.

Results: Usually available within two weeks.

Food Allergy Assay (IgG RAST and Food Antigen Immune Complex [FICA])

Type: Blood test.

Purpose: To diagnose food sensitivities and allergies. Many alcoholics are allergic to corn, wheat, and dairy products. A RAST is a radioallergosorbent test, a laboratory procedure that many family doctors now use in place of skin testing for food allergies. The most common RAST test for food allergies, the major #2 food panel, can detect allergies to thirty different foods, including milk, corn, wheat, egg white, chocolate, and soy. These so-called immediate reactors usually trigger allergies mediated by IgE, an immune-system component associated with such responses as hives, eczema, nausea, vomiting, and life-threatening anaphylactic shock. The food panel can also detect allergies that cause symptoms that may occur up to three days after the offending food is eaten. These can include headache, fatigue, and depression—symptoms you may not associate with something you ate within the past few days.

Where available: Your doctor can draw a blood sample and send it to any one of a number of laboratories that run this test. The one we use provides a sixteen-page personalized food-allergy printout and rotation diet, a cookbook, and a toll-free telephone number to call for free nutritional and dietary consultation.

Preparation required: None.

Results: Usually available in two weeks.

Hair Analysis

Type: Study of a hair sample.

Purpose: To detect deficiencies or toxic buildup of the following minerals, trace elements, and toxic metals: calcium, magnesium, zinc, copper, chromium, sodium, potassium, selenium, lead, nickel, cadmium, mercury, and arsenic.

Where available: Your doctor can send your hair sample to any of the laboratories listed in Appendix C. All have voluntarily accepted guidelines for hair element analysis established by the Hair Analysis Standardization Board of the American Holistic Medical Institute.

Preparations required: Simply snip a lock of your hair according to the following directions:

1. Do not submit dyed hair or hair that has a permanent wave less than one month old (a pubic-hair sample may be substituted for scalp hair).

2. Cut the hair as close to the scalp as possible and discard all but the first one and a half inches closest to the scalp.

3. If possible, clip the hair from the nape of your neck.

4. Place a total of one gram in a small envelope for submission. Your doctor can obtain a kit with a cardboard scale from the laboratory or you may choose to deal with the lab directly.

Results: Usually available in two weeks.

Note: Results will come with a printout detailing your mineral and toxic metal levels. These must be interpreted by a physician or nutritionist trained to appreciate the implications and to prescribe therapeutic doses to remedy any deficiencies or toxic buildups. Certain high readings may indicate storage of the mineral in question in the hair and soft tissues and an unavailability in blood and bone. Thus it is vital not to accept all the readings at face value (a sample of a hair-analysis test result appears in Figure 7 on page 153). The lab will provide duplicate copies of the results and the computerized analysis. Ask your doctor for these copies for your records.

Amino-Acid Analysis: Neuropsychiatric Panel

Type: Blood test.

Purpose: To measure plasma levels of various amino acids. Alcohol can destroy these natural chemicals, which can cause biochemical changes that prevent normal formation and function of neurotransmitters, the brain chemicals that underlie emotions, self-awareness, memory, and perception.

Where available: Your doctor can send your blood sample to any laboratory offering this test; we use Tyson and Associates in Hawthorne, California.

Preparation required: None.

Results: Usually available in two weeks.

Your completed charts plus your lab-test results will tell you whether or not alcohol has damaged you and, if so, in what way. Armed with this knowledge, you can design a personal treatment plan for biochemical restoration. The first step is a big one: breaking your addiction. Like most of our clients at HRC, you have probably tried to stop drinking many times in the past. I know you dread the misery of withdrawal. But this time will be different. I can't guarantee that you won't feel a few twinges, but I can tell you that most of HRC's clients are amazed at how easy withdrawal is with the aid of our special detoxification formula. I'm confident that you'll agree.

Week Two: Breaking the Addiction

I'm sure you're anxious to get started, and I know you're curious about that magic detoxification formula I mentioned at the end of the last chapter. Magic may be too strong a word but if you have tried to detoxify before—and failed—you're going to get the surprise of your life this week. You're going to be taking a lot of vitamins, minerals, and amino acids, up to sixty each day, in a formula designed to ease alcohol withdrawal symptoms and eliminate your cravings for alcohol. If you are typical of our HRC clients, you're going to feel terrific after your first weekend of taking the formula. Some of our clients feel so good that they tell me they don't need the rest of the program. My standard joke is that the detox formula is bad for business; when cravings for alcohol disappear, so do some new clients! Seriously, this formula works better than I dared dream. Our clients love it. I'll never forget a telephone call I got one morning.

"Do you remember me?" said the voice on the phone. "I saw you a year ago. I couldn't afford your program, but you gave me the detox formula." (I have done that occasionally for alcoholics who have been in and out of other treatment programs and are at the end of their rope financially and emotionally.)

"How are you doing?" I answered.

"Well, I took your detox formula for eight months, and I never drank the whole time! Then I went to California and lost the instructions. I'm back to alcohol now and can't get off. Do you think I could have another copy of that formula?"

I was shocked that he had taken the potent detox formula for such a long time, but evidently it had helped him enormously. Of course I saw him again. He still couldn't afford formal treatment, but he was certain he could do without alcohol once he resumed taking the detox formula.

Actually, we use two HRC detox formulas. Each is made up of the same nine supplements; the doses in formula 1 are a bit higher for reasons I will explain later. You will take the formula recommended for you for one week. A bit further on in this chapter you'll learn what each nutrient will do for you, which formula you should take, and why. But first, let's consider some of the realities and practicalities of detoxification.

Setting the Stage

Plan to get started over the weekend—most withdrawal symptoms that could develop will occur during this time. Most of our HRC clients feel well enough to go to work by Monday morning.

I have stressed before how important it is to have a companion's support while you are following this program. This is particularly true during the first few days of detoxification. If you live alone, ask a close friend or relative to spend the weekend with you.

If you are alone in a city of strangers, you can find instant support among the members of AA. Look in the telephone directory for the listing for AA or Intergroup. The essence of AA's philosophy is "let us love you until you can love yourself." AA members take that creed very seriously. Call Intergroup. Someone will be glad to help you. If no one else is available, please consider taking a physician into your confidence.

Your Alcohol Detox Profile

The next step is to determine which detox category best describes you so you can choose the plan that fits your needs. Circle the statements that are true in each category. Your answers will undoubtedly cluster in one of the four categories. Take the results of this test very seriously and detoxify only as instructed.

Category 1

1. You often have gone without alcohol for days (or longer).
2. You have never suffered a convulsion while withdrawing from alcohol.
3. You experience only slight to moderate shakiness, sleeplessness, heart palpitations, night sweats, or nervousness when you stop drinking.
4. You can and do function on the job without alcohol.

If most of the responses you checked fall under this heading, *you can detoxify alone.*

Category 2

1. You have been drinking regularly but occasionally cut back on amounts or skip a day of drinking without severe effects.
2. You have no history of convulsions when withdrawing from alcohol (or you are taking an anticonvulsant drug like Dilantin).
3. You experience withdrawal symptoms severe enough to warrant taking time off from work to detox.

If most of the responses you checked fall under this heading, *you can detox with the aid of a friend or relative.*

Category 3

1. You have suffered convulsions during previous attempts to detoxify from alcohol.*
2. You drink one quart of liquor or a twelve-pack of beer daily or when binging.
3. You experience marked withdrawal symptoms when detoxifying—tremors, heart palpitations, agitation. You may feel hyper and develop mild delirium.
4. Your blood pressure is higher than 160/100.
5. Your withdrawal symptoms are so severe that you must remain in bed while detoxifying.

If most of the responses you checked fall under this heading, *you can detox with the help of a friend or relative and medication, under a doctor's supervision.*

Category 4

1. You have major medical complications of alcoholism or a major psychiatric illness.
2. You are chronically alcoholic with a history of repeated grand mal seizures when withdrawing from alcohol as well as hallucinations or serious heart problems.

If either of these statements is true, *you MUST detox in a hospital under medical supervision.* Afterward, you can begin taking the detox formula. You will need it. You may be alcohol free when you complete an inpatient detox program, but since you will have accomplished little or no biochemical repair, you probably won't be feeling very good. The detox formula will reduce your cravings for alcohol and ease any lingering withdrawal symptoms. It will also begin the important job of restoring your nutritional well-being. You will be feeling better within days after you begin to take the detox formula.

---

*Your physician may prescribe the drug Dilantin to prevent convulsions and/or Librium to reduce anxiety and/or medication to reduce your blood pressure.

Play by the Rules to Assure Success

Now that you know how you'll detox, there are a few things you must do to prepare:

1. Remove all liquor from your living quarters, office, car, and wherever else you have stashed it. Don't argue. Do it!

2. Consider asking your doctor for a mild tranquilizer to ease withdrawal only if you have had difficulty in the past. Since drugs increase the toxins in your body, it is best to avoid them unless your doctor considers them necessary. At HRC we have found that BuSpar, an antianxiety drug available only by prescription, is very helpful. Unlike Valium or Librium, BuSpar is not addictive. If your doctor prescribes it, take 5 mg to 10 mg three times a day during detoxification.

3. If you have a history of convulsions when in alcohol withdrawal, ask your doctor to prescribe an anticonvulsant like Dilantin and be sure to fill your prescription *before* you begin the detox process. (Seizures rarely occur with the HRC detox formula because two of the nutrients it contains, magnesium and Efamol, have anticonvulsant effects.)

4. From now on, avoid all drinking parties, bars, and drinking buddies. I know this is tough, but if you continue to see drinkers, chances are good that they will persuade you to drink with them.

5. Don't change addictions by substituting caffeine and nicotine for alcohol.

6. Avoid foods containing refined sugars and white flour. Try to eat at least three meals a day even if your appetite is poor. Good food choices are fruits and vegetables, nuts and salads, fish, eggs, and chicken. Quantity is not as important as the nutritional quality of the foods you eat.

So What's the Formula?

The HRC detox formula (Table 2) combination of vitamins, minerals, amino acids, and other nutrients that has amazing power to cleanse the body of the effects of alcohol, eliminate cravings and dramatically reduce withdrawal symptoms. The detox formula also begins the all-important job of replacing the natural chemicals alcohol has destroyed and repairing the existing damage. The detox formula is based on the work of researchers from all over the world. The dosages have been tested and fine-tuned over the years, and the nutrients are readily available at most health-food stores and many drugstores.

Table 2. The HRC Detox Formula

Nutrient	Dose Each Capsule
Glutamine	500 mg
Free-form amino acids	750 mg
DL-Phenylalanine	500 mg
Tryptophan*	500 mg
Vitamin C	1000 mg
Calcium/Magnesium	300/150 mg
Efamol	500 mg
Multivitamin/mineral formula	(see Table 5)
Pancreatic enzymes	425 mg

*Use tryptophan only if the FDA lifts the current ban on its sale.

Which Detox Formula Is Best for You?

As I mentioned earlier, there are two versions of the detox formula (Tables 3 and 4). The only difference between them is that the nutrient doses in formula 2 are somewhat lower than those in formula 1.

Your alcohol biotype determines which detox formula you should use. If you do not clearly fit into a single biotype, start on detox formula 1. If you develop any stomach upset or nausea, switch to

Table 3. Detox Formula 1, Hourly Instructions

Upon rising (at least ½ hour before breakfast)	Glutamine—2 capsules Amino acids—3 capsules DL-Phenylalanine—1 capsule Vitamin C—3 capsules*
8:00 A.M. (breakfast)	Calcium/magnesium—3 capsules Efamol—3 capsules Multivitamin/mineral—2 capsules Pancreatic enzymes—2 capsules
10:00 A.M.	Vitamin C—3 capsules* 1000 mg capsules
12:00 noon (or ½ hour before lunch)	Glutamine—2 capsules Amino acids—3 capsules DL-Phenylalanine—1 capsule
1:00 P.M. (lunch)	Vitamin C—3 capsules* Calcium/magnesium—3 capsules Efamol—3 capsules Multivitamin/mineral—2 capsules Pancreatic enzymes—2 capsules
4:00 P.M.	Glutamine—2 capsules Amino acids—3 capsules DL-Phenylalanine—1 capsule Vitamin C—3 capsules*
6:00 P.M. (dinner)	Efamol—3 capsules Multivitamin/mineral—2 capsules Pancreatic enzymes—2 capsules
7:00 P.M.	Vitamin C—3 capsules*
10:00 P.M. (at bedtime)	Tryptophan—2–4 capsules† Vitamin C—3 capsules* Calcium/magnesium—3 capsules

*If diarrhea develops, cut dose in half.
†Use tryptophan only if the FDA lifts the current ban on its sale.

Table 4. Detox Formula 2, Hourly Instructions

Upon rising (at least ½ hour before breakfast)	Glutamine—2 capsules Amino acids—2 capsules DL-Phenylalanine—1 capsule Vitamin C—2 capsules*
8:00 A.M. (breakfast)	Calcium/magnesium—2 capsules Efamol—2 capsules Multivitamin/mineral—2 capsules Pancreatic enzymes—2 capsules
10:00 A.M.	Vitamin C—2 capsules* 1000 mg capsules
12:00 noon (or ½ hour before lunch)	Glutamine—2 capsules Amino acids—2 capsules DL-Phenylalanine—1 capsule
1:00 P.M. (lunch)	Vitamin C—2 capsules* Calcium/magnesium—2 capsules Efamol—2 capsules Multivitamin/mineral—2 capsules Pancreatic enzymes—2 capsules
4:00 P.M.	Glutamine—2 capsules Amino acids—2 capsules Vitamin C—2 capsules*
6:00 P.M. (dinner)	Efamol—2 capsules Multivitamin/mineral—2 capsules Pancreatic enzymes—2 capsules
7:00 P.M.	Vitamin C—2 capsules*
10:00 P.M. (at bedtime)	Tryptophan—2–4 capsules† Vitamin C—2 capsules* Calcium/magnesium—2 capsules

*If diarrhea develops, cut dose in half.
**Use tryptophan only if the FDA lifts the current ban on its sale.
†Use tryptophan only if the FDA lifts the current ban on its sale.

formula 2 on the second day and continue for the next six days. Find your biotype in the list below to see which formula you should use:

- II ADH/THIQ: Detox formula 1. Your superefficient dehydrogenase II liver enzymes can metabolize large amounts of drugs and are certainly up to the job of processing and absorbing the much-needed natural chemicals in the formula.

  Exception: Long-term chronic II ADH/THIQ drinkers who have some degree of liver damage should use detox formula 2. If you don't yet have the results of your lab tests, assume that you have liver damage if your high tolerance for alcohol has dropped dramatically and you now begin to feel uncomfortable or ill after only a few drinks. If so, you'll be better off using the less potent formula 2.
- Omega-6 EFA deficient: Detox formula 1.
- Allergic/Addicted: Detox formula 2. The dosages in this formula are somewhat lower to suit your more sensitive and reactive body chemistry.

Symptoms—if any—related to detoxification will be most intense during the first three days of the week. I have found that everyone reacts differently. Some of our clients have no problems at all. Others tell us that they feel a little shaky, tired, and irritable. Overall, however, expect only a minimum of discomfort.

Is the Formula Safe?

Absolutely! The natural chemicals it contains belong in your body. They are not toxic the way drugs are. Indeed, compared to drugs, nutrient therapy is unbelievably safe. Comparisons of reports of toxicity and deaths compiled by the American Association of Poison Control Centers from 1983 to 1987 show that there were NO deaths as a result of nutritional therapy but 1,132 deaths caused by prescription drugs *used correctly* and another 337 caused by aspirin and similar painkillers.

Practical Advice for Managing Your Nutrients

The nutrients used at HRC are the best quality we can find. They are in capsules rather than the difficult-to-digest hard-pressed tablets. For information about obtaining the HRC DETOX FORMULA and all other formulas appearing in this book, you can call BIO-RECOVERY at 1-800-24 SOBER.

Take your first round of amino acids when you wake up.

If you are working, the easiest way to keep your detox nutrients on hand is to package each day's supply in four small plastic bags:

1 and 2. Package your prelunch and predinner amino acids in two separate bags. Each should contain glutamine, free-form amino acids, and DL-phenylalanine.

Use one package one-half hour before lunch and the other at the end of the working day just before you head home to supper.

3. Carry your vitamin C in a separate plastic bag. You will take a dose at 7:00 A.M., 10:00 A.M., 1:00 P.M., 4:00 P.M., 7:00 P.M., and 10:00 P.M. You will probably be taking three of these doses during working hours.

4. The fourth bag should contain your lunchtime doses of your remaining nutrients: Calcium/magnesium, Efamol, multivitamin/mineral formula, and pancreatic enzymes.

Contents of the Detox Formula

On the following pages, I'll give you a full description of the contents of the detox formula. I want you to know what you are taking and why it is so important that you swallow so many capsules. You will see that wherever there is the slightest possibility that a nutrient could have any adverse effect, I have included specific precautions.

Your local health store stocks the components of the detox formula. Be sure the products you buy are hypoallergenic (their coatings or binders contain no sugar, wheat, dairy, or corn). In Appendix C, you'll find a list of companies whose products conform to HRC specifications.

Be sure to buy everything you need for your detox formula before you begin detoxing.

Vitamin C (Ascorbic Acid)

Research suggesting that vitamin C can reverse addictive states dates back to 1958, when studies found that injecting vitamin C greatly reduced or abolished the narcotic effects of morphine in addicted rats. But it wasn't until 1977 that researchers Alfred Libby and Irwin W. Stone published the first study of the effect of vitamin C on human drug addicts.

One of their case histories described how vitamin C reversed incoherence in a teenager on angel dust (PCP) in half an hour. In a subsequent study, Libby and Stone intravenously administered twenty-five to eighty-five grams of vitamin C (accompanied by other essential vitamins and minerals) daily to heroin addicts. No withdrawal symptoms developed. "Should a fix [heroin] be taken, it is immediately detoxified and no 'high' is produced," the researchers reported.

Vitamin C has the same effect on alcoholics. In fact, in 1985 Libby received a U.S. patent for his method of detoxifying alcoholics and drug addicts with a combination of vitamin C, calcium, magnesium, and thiamine. Today, many nutritionally oriented practitioners use Libby's method to detoxify patients from alcohol and other drugs.

Is it safe? Without a doubt, vitamin C is one of the least toxic substances known. Nobel Prize–winning scientist Linus Pauling tells us that people have ingested 125 grams at one time without harm and notes that while it has been suggested that a high intake of vitamin C can cause kidney stones, "not a single case of such kidney stones exists in medical literature."

The HRC detox formula that we infuse at entry to treatment intravenously contains sixty to seventy-five grams of sodium ascorbate (ascorbate is the same thing as ascorbic acid, or vitamin C), combined with calcium and magnesium. Of course, you won't be giving yourself infusions. But taking megadoses of vitamin C by mouth will go a long way toward reducing your cravings for alcohol and preventing or lessening withdrawal symptoms.

Some advice about taking vitamin C:

- Buy the kind that has been buffered (alkalized) with sodium, calcium and magnesium, or potassium. It's easier on your stomach. The hypoallergenic vitamin C we use at HRC is made from sago palm, not corn, and comes from Allergy Research Group in San Leandro, California.

• If you continue taking large amounts of vitamin C by mouth, eventually you will experience some diarrhea. When you do, begin to reduce your dose by one-third to one-half, or space the doses an hour further apart. The diarrhea almost always stops when the dose is cut in half. If it continues, stop taking vitamin C to see if it is causing the problem. In rare cases, diarrhea can be an ongoing health problem in alcoholics, but this is not related to taking vitamin C.

Calcium/Magnesium

These minerals also dramatically reduce many withdrawal symptoms. Alcoholics excrete great amounts of both calcium and magnesium in their urine: twenty minutes after drinking one ounce of alcohol, urinary calcium output increases by 100 percent, magnesium by 167 percent.

During detoxification, inadequate calcium levels can cause painful leg cramps, insomnia, nervousness, slow reflexes, and emotional instability.

A magnesium deficiency interferes with your ability to sleep and can make you irritable, depressed, and dizzy. It can also cause muscle tremors, high blood pressure, and changes in heart rhythm. The severe deficiencies we sometimes see in alcoholics can cause convulsive seizures accompanied by delirium. Immediate magnesium replacement is critical. Researcher E. B. Flink, M.D., of the University of Virginia, has found that hallucinations, uncontrollable tremors, inability to sleep, and a sort of waking tremor occur only among alcoholics with severely depleted magnesium stores. These symptoms may be masked while you're drinking, but you'll notice them when you stop. The magnesium in the detox formula reduces or eliminates these symptoms.

If you buy calcium and magnesium separately, be sure that each calcium citrate tablet contains 300 milligrams of calcium and each magnesium oxide tablet 150 milligrams of magnesium.

Amino Acids

Amino acids are the chief components of protein. Normally, they are extracted from food. Some are converted into the brain chemicals (neurotransmitters) that control moods, memory, and feelings. Alcoholics and drug addicts are often so depleted of amino acids that the conversion process slows or stops, which causes depression, poor recall, hostile and aggressive behavior, mental confusion, anxiety, and paranoia.

The HRC detox formula contains Aminoplex, a combination of eighteen amino acids in their purest forms. For best absorption, these capsules should be taken on an empty stomach.

Warning: If you have systemic lupus erythematosus, are on methadone therapy, or have certain rare inborn genetic errors in amino-acid metabolism, do not take amino acids except under a doctor's supervision.

In addition to the amino-acid combination, you will be taking large, separate doses of two, possibly three, amino acids. The two are glutamine and DL-phenylalanine. The third is tryptophan, which, at this writing, is banned from the market in the United States by the Food and Drug Administration. (Since the ban probably will be lifted soon, I'll tell you all about tryptophan, how it can help you, and why it is not currently available.) Let's start this discussion with an amino acid that you'll bless whenever alcoholic cravings develop.

Glutamine

This amino acid has a truly amazing ability to reduce cravings for alcohol. In a study reported in the *Quarterly Journal of Studies on Alcohol,* the desire to drink was significantly diminished among alcoholics who took glutamine, while cravings continued unabated among a comparison group who received a placebo. The alcoholics who took glutamine also reported that they were less anxious and able to sleep better.

I have noticed that HRC clients complain of a return of cravings within forty-eight hours when they neglect to refill their glutamine supplies. You can quench a sudden desire for alcohol by opening a 500-milligram glutamine capsule and letting it dissolve in your mouth.

(Substances placed under the tongue are absorbed directly into the bloodstream and take effect immediately.) Glutamine is one of our clients' favorite nutrients.

DL-Phenylalanine

Phenylalanine, an essential amino acid, is needed for formation of the neurotransmitters called catecholamines, which include dopamine, norepinephrine, and epinephrine. It is also a constituent of a number of brain hormones. During detox, DL-phenylalanine reduces physical pain and combats mental fatigue. It comes in 500-milligram capsules.

D-phenylalanine contributes to this effect by blocking the breakdown of endorphins, potent natural painkillers and mood elevators, in the central nervous system.

L-phenylalanine is converted into norepinephrine, an excitatory neurotransmitter, creating an antidepressant effect.

Warning: Do not use phenylalanine if you take MAO inhibitors for depression or suffer from any of the following conditions: phenylketonuria (PKU), hepatic cirrhosis, melanoma, or migraine headaches.

Niacin, vitamin B_6, copper, vitamin C, iron, and folic acid must be present for proper metabolism of phenylalanine. The detox formula contains all of them.

L-Tryptophan

You may remember all the publicity surrounding the removal of tryptophan from the market. The FDA acted after several deaths and a number of illnesses were traced to contaminated batches of the nutrient from Japan. The investigation of the exact nature of the chemical contaminant responsible has been completed, but so far there has been no indication of when the FDA will permit reintroduction of tryptophan. This is unfortunate for alcoholics who desperately need to replace tryptophan to resume normal sleep and alleviate alcohol-induced anxiety and depression. Although tryptophan is important to recovery, *do not* take any that was purchased before the FDA ordered it removed from the market. However, on the assumption that the FDA will eventually lift the ban, I'll describe tryptophan and its benefits. When 500-milligram capsules become available again, you can add it to your detox formula.

The brain uses tryptophan to produce the neurotransmitter serotonin, which maintains emotional calm, regulates sleep, and prevents depression. Suicidal patients show significant decreases in serotonin levels, and autopsies have shown that a very low brain level of serotonin is the one biological marker of suicide. People who are depressed or agitated can often use tryptophan as effectively as antidepressants.

Research has shown that alcoholic blackouts are caused by insufficient levels of tryptophan. Since most alcoholics suffer blackouts, it makes sense to assume that insufficient tryptophan is to blame and that it also underlies any depression and sleeplessness they are experiencing.

To convert tryptophan to serotonin, your body must have adequate levels of the following nutrients: folic acid, vitamin B_6, magnesium, and niacin, as well as glutamine. The detox formula provides them all.

Efamol

This is a trade name for oil of evening primrose, the only nutritional source of an oil needed for formation of prostaglandin E_1, an important brain metabolite. Normally, our bodies convert linolenic acid from food into a body chemical called gamma-linolenic acid (GLA) which, in turn, forms prostaglandin E_1 (PGE_1). Since alcohol disrupts this conversion process, you need Efamol as a source of vital GLA.

Efamol can reduce alcohol withdrawal symptoms and improve mental processes. A study (E. Glen et al.) comparing two groups of alcoholics in the process of detoxifying found withdrawal symptoms were minimal and mental processes much improved only among the group that took Efamol. Several studies in animals have confirmed that prostaglandin E_1 can prevent alcohol withdrawal syndrome. Replacing prostaglandin E_1 can also prevent central-nervous-system impairment and liver damage. Because it has anticonvulsant properties, PGE_1 also protects against seizures.

When Efamol—in 500-milligram dosages—was added to our HRC detox formula, we noticed that patients' withdrawal symptoms were far less severe than they had been without it.

Multivitamin / Mineral Formula

Alcoholics are often deficient in vitamins and minerals because of poor nutrition and poor absorption of needed nutrients. At HRC we use a multivitamin formula (Multi Vi-Min) developed by the Allergy Research Group in San Leandro, California, to replace missing nutrients (Table 5). The formula contains no yeast, wheat, corn, soy, dairy products, preservatives, or chemical dilutants. The most hypoallergenic forms of inorganic minerals are used.

The B Complex in the Multivitamin/Mineral Formula:

Depletion of these vitamins dramatically undermines brain and nervous system stability. A number of studies have shown that rats can be transformed from teetotalers into alcoholics by taking the B vitamins out of their diets. Their preference for alcohol gradually disappears as the vitamins are restored; when vitamin levels return to normal, the rats refuse alcohol and drink only water. Because they are so important, you should know more about the B vitamins:

- Thiamine (vitamin B_1): Alcohol blocks thiamine absorption, causing neurological and mental symptoms including memory loss, central-nervous-system damage, numbness and tingling in the arms and legs, mental confusion, nervousness, headache, and poor concentration. It is responsible for Wernicke-Korsakoff syndrome, the irreversible brain deterioration that can occur in the later stages of alcoholism.
- Niacin (vitamin B_3): Abram Hoffer, M.D., a pioneer in niacin research, notes that the symptoms of anxiety neurosis are strikingly similar to those of mild niacin deficiency (subclincial pellagra): depression, fatigue, apprehension, headache, hyperactivity, and insomnia. AA cofounder Bill Wilson discovered the benefits of niacin replacement therapy for himself and published three communications to AA physicians that summarized research supporting niacin's many benefits for alcoholics. Russell Smith, M.D., nephew of AA cofounder Bob Smith, also contributed to the research. His studies of the long-term effect of niacin supplements showed that cravings were reduced, feelings of well-

Table 5. HRC Multivitamin/Mineral Formula

Nutrient	1 Capsule	6 Capsules
Vitamin A (palmitate)	4,000 IU	24,000 IU
Vitamin B_1 (thiamine)	20 mg	120 mg
Vitamin B_2 (riboflavin)	10 mg	60 mg
Vitamin B_3 (niacinamide)	30 mg	180 mg
Vitamin B_5 (pantothenic acid)	100 mg	600 mg
Vitamin B_6 (pyridoxine)	30 mg	180 mg
Pyridoxal-5'-phosphate	1 mg	6 mg
Vitamin B_{12} (cobalamine)	80 mcg	480 mcg
Folic acid	60 mcg	360 mcg
Biotin	80 mcg	480 mcg
PABA (para-aminobenzoic acid)	40 mg	240 mg
Vitamin E (DL-alpha-tocopherol acetate)	80 IU	480 IU
Calcium (dicalcium phosphate)	50 mg	300 mg
Magnesium (magnesium oxide)	50 mg	300 mg
Potassium (potassium chloride)	20 mg	120 mg
Manganese (manganese sulfate)	3 mg	18 mg
Zinc (zinc sulfate)	5.7 mg	34.2 mg
Copper (copper sulfate)	300 mcg	1.8 mg
Selenium (sodium selenite)	40 mcg	240 mcg
Vanadium (vanadium pentoxide)	40 mcg	240 mcg
Molybdenum (sodium molybdate)	40 mcg	240 mcg
Glutamic acid	40 mg	240 mg
Chromium	80 mcg	480 mcg
Iron (ammonium ferric citrate)	3.6 mg	21.6 mg

being increased, energy improved, and moods stabilized among 87 percent of the chronic alcoholics participating in his study. Surprisingly, the alcoholics studied also reported that they lost their former tolerance for high amounts of alcohol.

- Pyridoxine (vitamin B_6): Vitamin B_6 is needed for formation of fifty different enzymes and is essential for the metabolism of all the amino acids and their conversion into neurotransmitters. We also need B_6 to maintain a stable immune system. Deficiencies are common among alcoholics. Symptoms include anxiety, nervousness, and depression. A severe deficiency can bring on convulsions, heightened anxiety, and extreme nervous exhaustion.

- Folic acid: Symptoms of deficiency include agitation, moodiness, headaches, depression, and fatigue; folic-acid deficiency also accounts for the decreased sex drive of heavy drinkers.

- Vitamin B_{12}: Depletion impairs concentration and memory and causes a stuporous type of depression and a number of mental disorders, including insanity.

- Choline and inositol: These B vitamins are essential for repair of alcohol-induced liver damage. Inositol also acts as a mild tranquilizer; choline improves learning capacity and memory.

- Pantothenic acid: This nutrient combats stress. In one study, prison volunteers fed a diet deficient in pantothenic acid became increasingly depressed, irritable, tense, dizzy, sullen, and quarrelsome. All symptoms disappeared when the nutrient was resupplied.

Pancreatic Enzymes

Heavy alcohol use disturbs the function of the pancreas, blocking the release of the enzymes needed to properly absorb and utilize nutrients. A few capsules of pancreatic enzymes will insure that you fully absorb the nutrients in the detox formula. (Pancreas, 700-mg, Allergy Research Group.)

Some Last Thoughts Before You Begin

As you prepare to detoxify and then move on to complete your repair program, please reach out to friends and relatives for support. We all need someone who cares about us. If your drinking buddies are your entire support team, you're headed for trouble. New friendships await you in AA or Women for Sobriety. Don't neglect these valuable resources. They are available nationwide.

It is also important not to underrate your emotional involvement with alcohol. It plays a powerful, seductive role in your life. To succeed in freeing your life from alcohol, you must provide some emotional safeguards for yourself. You should find some new friends or revive your ties to old friends you may have lost touch with while you were drinking. You should also begin to think about new activities to fill the time you spent drinking. One of the most rewarding investments for those extra hours is to begin a program of exercise. Consider starting with a minimum of half an hour daily of brisk walking, or join a friend for cycling, swimming, skating, or whatever you used to enjoy before drinking robbed you of those pleasures. Whatever you do, don't leave a void. Remember, loneliness and boredom can sabotage your recovery.

As you begin, bear in mind two AA affirmations that have helped millions achieve and maintain sobriety:

One day at a time.
Easy does it.

This kind of self-talk can help you through any shaky hours ahead. What you tell yourself during this critical period can make an enormous difference to your success or failure. Think positively. You won't be disappointed.

Seven

Week Three:
Correcting Chemistry

Are you ready for the main event? By the time you read this chapter you should have completed or almost completed your week-long detox plan. If so, you are already beginning to feel better. You have seen for yourself what the nutrients in the formula can do to ease the misery of alcohol withdrawal. You're probably beginning to understand and appreciate the power of these natural chemicals to restore your health.

The best is yet to come. During the next four weeks you're going to repair the biochemical damage alcohol has caused. Perhaps for the first time in years you'll begin to feel strong, energetic, and healthy in body and mind. You will join the ranks of the hundreds of HRC clients who tell me that this program has not only restored their health but has enabled them to reassert control over their lives. They are free of cravings for alcohol and free of the negative emotions that drove them to drink.

After you have been on the detox formula *one week,* you will continue your seven-week program by cutting back on the high level of nutrients you were taking. To the adjusted nutrient plan levels you are going to add some new ones to improve your general health and to help bring your wayward blood sugar under control. You are also going to begin a healthy new diet filled with a tempting variety of wonderful fresh foods and free of refined sugars and other junk foods that have contributed to your problems with alcohol.

If you are typical of our HRC clients, you are among the 80 to 95 percent of alcoholics who are hypoglycemic. As you will learn on the pages ahead, hypoglycemia—low blood sugar—usually underlies and complicates alcoholism. Correcting this metabolic disorder is as important to recovery as restoring the nutrients alcohol has depleted.

Even if you have not had the lab tests recommended in Chapter 4, you can safely assume that you are at least somewhat hypoglycemic and are suffering from the effects of depleted or unavailable natural nutrients. You can't go wrong making these assumptions. Most alcoholics are affected on both counts. And in any case, neither the nutrients nor the diet contained in this chapter can possibly hurt you. They can only enhance your health and well-being.

The job of correcting your body chemistry begins with the adjusted nutrient plan, a slightly different combination of the vitamins and minerals you have been taking in your detox formula.

Your Cruising Speed

In Tables 6 and 7, you'll find the appropriate adjusted nutrient plan for your alcohol biotype. Look over your list carefully. You will see that it contains all the nutrients you took during detox plus two newcomers, the antioxidant formula and fortified flax. Both can help improve and protect your health.

Antioxidant Complex

These capsules contain a combination of beta-carotene (vitamin A), vitamin C, zinc, selenium, the polypeptide glutathione, the amino acids methionine and cysteine, vitamin E, dimethylglycine, as well as ubiquinone (coenzyme Q-10) and lipoic acid. These substances are antioxidants, which can help prevent harmful reactions in the body that can lead to heart attack, stroke, cataract, cancer, and arthritis. The same reactions are also involved in the aging process. They involve oxidation, a sort of rusting at the cellular level. The substances in the antioxidant formula can prevent oxidation and slow reactions already in progress. They also inhibit the action of free radicals, unstable molecules that can inflict damage at the cellular level, thus causing disease.

Antioxidants also protect you against the cellular damage from such environmental pollutants as cigarette smoke and automobile exhaust as well as the potentially carcinogenic effect of drugs, food dyes, chemicals, and other toxins. The antioxidant formula we use at HRC is from Ecological Formulas, Concord, California.

Fortified Flax

This is an excellent source of the omega-3 essential fatty acid (EFA) needed for formation of our steroid hormones. Omega-3 is also needed for proper immune-system functioning and the nerve-circuit activation that affects thinking and moods. It also helps regulate body temperature and serves as the messenger for hormone secretion and uptake of B vitamins. Because of the way our food is processed, your diet probably is pretty low in omega-3, unless you eat a lot of fresh fish.

The fortified flax used at HRC is from OMEGA-Life, Inc., Brookfield, Wisconsin.

Your Present Inability to Absorb

There is an important reason why you must continue to take such big doses of the nutrients you need. At this point, your ability to absorb these vital natural chemicals is poor. Researchers H. Tao and H. Fox have found that early in the recovery process, alcoholics excrete through their urine most of a B vitamin (pantothenic acid) they took. This occurs even when deficiencies exist. The only way to overcome this malabsorption problem is to temporarily supply megadoses of the nutrients needed. This way, your body will pick up some traces despite your damaged ability to absorb.

Keeping Track of What You Take

At this point, you must be wondering how in the world you are going to keep track of all these pills. Relax. It isn't as hard as you think. In Tables 6 and 7, you will find adjusted nutrient plans for each alcohol biotype. The lists are very easy to follow and will enable you to keep an accurate record of what you're taking and when. You may want to make several copies of your list and keep one in your purse or wallet, another at work, and another in the bathroom or kitchen at home—wherever you keep your supply of nutrients.

Table 6. Adjusted Nutrient Plan for II ADH/THIQ and Omega-6 EFA Deficient Biotypes

Upon rising (at least ½ hour before breakfast)	Glutamine—2 capsules Amino acids—2 capsules DL-Phenylalanine—1 capsule
8:00 A.M. (breakfast)	Vitamin C—2 capsules* Calcium/magnesium—2 capsules Efamol—2 capsules Multivitamin/mineral—3 capsules Pancreatic enzymes—2 capsules Antioxidant complex—1 capsule Fortified flax—2 tablespoons in juice or applesauce

Table 6. Adjusted Nutrient Plan for II ADH/THIQ and Omega-6
EFA Deficient Biotypes (Continued)

11:30 A.M. (or at least ½ hour before lunch)	Glutamine—2 capsules Amino Acids—2 capsules DL-Phenylalanine—1 capsule	Package together for work
12:00 noon (lunch)	Vitamin C—2 capsules* Efamol—2 capsules Pancreatic enzymes—2 capsules	Package together for work
4:30 P.M.	Glutamine—2 capsules Amino acids—2 capsules DL-Phenylalanine, 1 capsule	Package together for work
6:00 P.M. (dinner)	Vitamin C—2 capsules* Efamol—2 capsules Multivitamin/mineral—3 capsules Pancreatic enzymes—2 capsules	
10:00 P.M. (at bedtime)	Tryptophan—2–4 capsules† Calcium/magnesium—2 capsules	

*If diarrhea develops, cut dose in half.
†Use tryptophan only if the FDA lifts the current ban on its sale.

Table 7. Adjusted Nutrient Plan for the
Allergic/Addicted Biotype

Upon rising (at least ½ hour before breakfast)	Glutamine—2 capsules Amino acids—1 capsule DL-Phenylalanine—1 capsule	
8:00 A.M. (breakfast)	Vitamin C—2 capsules* Calcium/magnesium—2 capsules Efamol—2 capsules Multivitamin/mineral—3 capsules Pancreatic enzymes—2 capsules Antioxidant complex—1 capsule Fortified flax—2 tablespoons in juice or applesauce	
11:30 A.M. (or ½ hour before lunch)	Glutamine—2 capsules Amino acids—2 capsules DL-Phenylalanine—1 capsule	Package together for work
12:00 noon (lunch)	Vitamin C—2 capsules* Pancreatic enzymes—2 capsules	Package together for work
4:30 P.M.	Glutamine—2 capsules Amino acids—1 capsule	Package together for work

**Table 7. Adjusted Nutrient Plan for the
Allergic/Addicted Biotype** (*Continued*)

6:00 P.M. (dinner)	Vitamin C—2 capsules* Efamol—2 capsules Multivitamin/mineral— 3 capsules Pancreatic enzymes—2 capsules
10:00 P.M. (at bedtime)	Tryptophan—2–4 capsules† Calcium/magnesium— 2 capsules

*If diarrhea develops, cut dose in half.
†Use tryptophan only if the FDA lifts the current ban on its sale.

Now let's tackle another major obstacle to recovery: hypoglycemia. If you have any doubts that your blood-sugar fluctuations influence the way you have been feeling physically and emotionally, you will soon see the connection.

Hypoglycemia and Alcoholism: What Research Shows

AA cofounder Bill Wilson was very interested in the link between alcoholism and hypoglycemia. He collected research papers demonstrating the extent of abnormal glucose fluctuations among alcoholics and sent three different reports on the subject to AA physicians. Wilson's interest was personal as well as professional. For many years, he suffered from depression and other hypoglycemic symptoms. He also consumed huge amounts of sugar and caffeine. Finally, by eliminating sugar and caffeine and making other dietary changes, he stabilized his blood sugar and achieved a sense of well-being.

Study after study has demonstrated that the vast majority of alcoholics are hypoglycemic. In one conducted by J. Poulos, D. Stafford, and K. Carron, fifty outpatient alcoholics and fifty halfway house alcoholics were compared with a control group of one hundred nurses and teenagers. Of the one hundred alcoholics, ninety-six proved to be hypoglycemic; only fourteen of the nonalcoholic controls were hypoglycemic. A three-year study by Robert Meiers, M.D., in Santa Cruz, California, found that more than 95 percent of alcoholics studied suffered from low blood sugar.

More evidence comes from Kenneth Williams, M.D., an internist at the University of Pittsburgh School of Medicine and a member of the national board of trustees of AA. Williams has found that a vast majority of his sober alcoholic patients are hypoglycemic; many have told him that their hypoglycemia had been diagnosed even before they started drinking.

Researcher and author Emanuel Cheraskin, M.D., found on the basis of six-hour glucose tolerance tests that between 75 and 90 percent of alcoholics studied were hypoglycemic. "Too much therapeutic emphasis has been placed on psychological factors," says Cheraskin, "while more basic biochemical deficiencies and defects in body chemistry have received relatively little attention."

These studies confirm the findings and views of endocrinologist John Tintera, M.D. After years of research, Tintera concluded that even recovered alcoholics who have been sober for many years continue to suffer the effects of hypoglycemia. He strongly believes that the treatment of alcoholism "centers essentially about control [of hypoglycemia] . . . by far the most important part of the physiological treatment of alcoholics is the complete restriction of easily absorbed carbohydrates."

Until their severe fluctuations in blood sugar are stabilized, Tintera warns that alcoholics will be predisposed to depression and what only appear to be "deep-rooted emotional or psychiatric disorders."

Tintera and other researchers who have documented the close connection between alcoholism and hypoglycemia consider psychoanalytic treatment "utterly unsuccessful [in rehabilitating alcoholics] since the deep-rooted emotional factor is, in reality, physiologically based."

Unfortunately, despite the work of Tintera and many others, few physicians today have a good understanding of hypoglycemia. Some may refuse your request for testing as unnecessary or even dismiss hypoglycemia as a fad disease. Others will test you but misinterpret the results because of the wide variance in diagnostic approaches practiced during the last two decades. For these reasons, you may need to search out a physician who fully appreciates the impact of hypoglycemia on alcoholism and can diagnose the condition accurately. If you haven't contacted a physician recommended by the organizations listed on pages 65–66, you may want to do so now.

Glucose Patterns in HRC Clients

The reason I'm so sure you are hypoglycemic is that during the past ten years I have found that the overwhelming majority at HRC suffer from this disorder. In our study of one hundred randomly selected clients, 88 percent proved to be hypoglycemic. Figure 4 shows glucose tolerance test patterns found among them. Figure 5 gives a breakdown of the types of hypoglycemic curves seen among these one hundred clients. (The sawtooth curve is not shown in Figure 6.) Ten percent demonstrated a sawtooth pattern of seesawing insulin and adrenaline release throughout the test after their initial hypoglycemic drop below fasting levels.

Hypoglycemic Symptoms

Are any of the symptoms in Table 8 familiar to you? This list was compiled by Stephen Gyland, M.D., on the basis of his study of twelve hundred hypoglycemic patients. Dr. Gyland himself experienced many of these symptoms; at one point, he became so incapacitated that he had to stop practicing medicine. In his futile search for help, he consulted physicians at a number of U.S. medical centers, including the famed Mayo Clinic. Finally, he pieced together the correct diagnosis of hypoglycemia, which he then verified by a six-hour glucose tolerance test. (I mention both five- and six-hour glucose tolerance tests in this book. The six-hour test is more thorough, but for most people, the five-hour version is sufficient.)

Figure 4. Glucose Tolerance Test Patterns
of HRC Clients at Entry

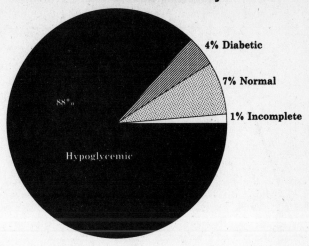

4% Diabetic

7% Normal

1% Incomplete

88%

Hypoglycemic

Figure 5. Hypoglycemic Curves
of HRC Clients

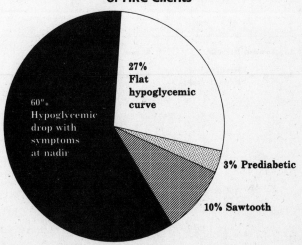

27%
Flat
hypoglycemic
curve

60%
Hypoglycemic
drop with
symptoms
at nadir

3% Prediabetic

10% Sawtooth

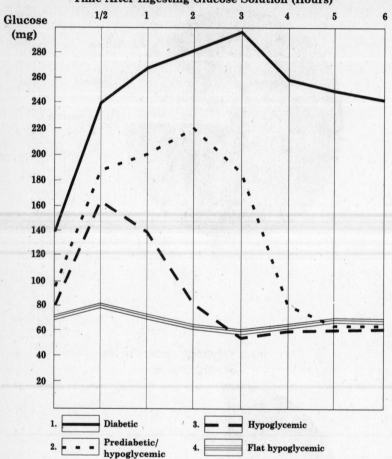

Figure 6. Six-Hour Glucose Tolerance Test

Time After Ingesting Glucose Solution (Hours)

Glucose (mg)

1. ▬▬▬ Diabetic
2. ▪ ▪ ▪ Prediabetic/ hypoglycemic
3. ▬ ▬ ▬ Hypoglycemic
4. ≡≡≡ Flat hypoglycemic

Table 8. Symptoms Reported
by Hypoglycemics

Symptom	Frequency
Nervousness	94%
Irritability	89%
Exhaustion	87%
Faintness, dizziness, tremors, cold sweats	86%
Depression	86%
Vertigo, dizziness	77%
Drowsiness	73%
Headaches	72%
Digestive disturbances	71%
Forgetfulness	69%
Insomnia	67%
Constant worrying; unprovoked anxieties	62%
Confusion	57%
Internal trembling	57%
Heart palpitations, rapid pulse	54%
Muscle pains	53%
Numbness	51%
Asocial or antisocial behavior	47%
Indecisiveness	50%
Crying spells	46%
Lack of sex drive (women)	44%
Allergies	43%
Incoordination	43%
Leg cramps	43%
Lack of concentration	42%
Blurred vision	40%

Table 8. Symptoms Reported
by Hypoglycemics *(Continued)*

Symptom	Frequency
Muscle twitching and jerking	40%
Itching and crawling skin sensations	39%
Gasping for breath	37%
Smothering spells	34%
Staggering	34%
Sighing and yawning	30%
Impotence (men)	29%
Unconsciousness	27%
Nightmares, night terrors	27%
Rheumatoid arthritis	24%
Phobias, fears	23%
Neurodermatitis	21%
Suicidal intent	20%
Nervous breakdown	17%
Convulsions	2%

The Hypoglycemic Cycle

To understand how these symptoms develop, you have to know something about glucose metabolism. Our bodies immediately convert foods high in refined sugar, white flour, or starch to blood sugar or glucose (the terms are interchangeable). When too much sugar builds up in the bloodstream, the pancreas pumps out extra insulin to counteract the overload.

If you are hypoglycemic and alcoholic, your oversensitized pancreas tries to control your excessive intake of both alcohol sugars and refined sugars. You overproduce insulin, which then removes too much sugar from your bloodstream. As a result, your blood sugar falls too far below normal levels. When it does, you may develop headaches and become irritable, anxious, fearful, tired, dizzy, confused, uncoordinated, forgetful, and unable to concentrate. You may feel and act antisocial.

Eventually, the physical stress produced by low blood sugar prompts an outpouring of the adrenal hormone epinephrine, which signals the liver to release emergency sugar (glycogen) to prevent further insulin shock. This can bring on other unpleasant reactions. You may feel shaky, weak, and sweaty, and you may be aware of a rapid heartbeat. You may have noticed that caffeine can produce these symptoms. It also stimulates the adrenal glands to trigger the release of stored glycogen to temporarily raise blood-sugar levels.

Blood sugar can also drop in response to a meal high in refined carbohydrates. This so-called postprandial fed-state hypoglycemia is very common among alcoholics and produces tremendous cravings for coffee and sweets. A study published in 1976 in the *Annals of the New York Academy of Sciences* reported that affected alcoholics are prone to "headache, weakness, tachycardia, hunger, excessive sweating, loss of concentration and anxiety. This type of hypoglycemia . . . can trigger further drinking to ease distressing symptoms and may lead to a syndrome described as the 'buildup to drink' . . . Many patients have apparently returned to alcohol usage during their rehabilitation programs because alcohol as a sugar and sedative drug alleviates many of the symptoms outlined above."

Postprandial hypoglycemia can also trigger psychological symptoms. When researcher F. Hale, M.D., administered glucose tolerance tests to sixty-seven subjects, mental stability, clarity, and agility were seriously affected among those whose glucose levels fell below sixty milligrams per deciliter. Dr. Hale concluded that "mental confusion does occur with postprandial hypoglycemia" and suggested that patients who complain of fatigue or depression two to four hours after meals have their blood sugar evaluated by a five-hour glucose tolerance test.

The Role of the Adrenals

Over time, the frequent outpouring of epinephrine (adrenaline) to prevent insulin shock takes a toll on your adrenal glands, your buffer against stress. When exhausted by continuing demands for adrenaline, they no longer have the strength to respond properly. This condition, called hypoadrenocorticism, interferes with or destroys the ability of the adrenals to protect you from stress. It also causes emotional instability.

Dr. Tintera believes that weakened adrenal protection plus heavy drinking are the primary factors leading to alcoholism:

Persons manifesting this genetic influence characteristically show a decreased metabolism, marked hypotension [low blood pressure] and a fondness or real craving for salt and carbohydrates . . .

[Many alcoholics] refer to their progressive candy binges, which incidentally induced greater adrenal involvement. Our alcoholic patients furthermore state that these binges lifted them from depression to a temporary period of well-being. Very soon, however, they discovered that emotional depression could be alleviated more effectively with alcohol. But this respite from depression and craving was of short duration so that continued drinking seemed the only answer. This craving is a physiologic attempt to increase the subject's blood sugar.

In the alcoholic, whether active or recovered, the prevailing factor is hypoglycemia. All the personality characteristics common to patients with hypoadrenocorticism (weakened adrenals) can be attributed to this hypoglycemia. They are aggravated in the addictive drinker and persist even in the (recovered) alcoholic.

The Dry-Drunk Syndrome = Masked Hypoglycemia

In an attempt to explain these hypoglycemic symptoms as a psychological phenomenon, mental-health professionals have developed an elaborate concept called the dry-drunk syndrome. This has been defined by M. Wellman, Ph.D., as a composite of "late withdrawal symptoms that include irritability, depression, insomnia, fatigue, restlessness, a sense of aloneness and distractibility." This exponent of the dry-drunk theory has noted that "a severe case mimics the physical signs of drunkenness." Abstinent alcoholics suffering from these symptoms have been advised to combat them by attending AA meetings, contacting AA members, and engaging in activities that keep their thoughts away from alcohol. Prayer and psychiatric help have also been recommended.

A Hazelden Foundation publication on the subject characterizes a typical dry-drunk alcoholic as grandiose, judgmental, impulsive, childish, easily distracted, and disorganized.

Another researcher, E. M. Jellinek, Ph.D., defines the dry-drunk syndrome as a manifestation of late withdrawal symptoms, which he views as "indications of insufficient adaptation on the symbolic level to an alcohol-free life."

These highfalutin psychological explanations ignore the fact that the symptoms are caused by a physical condition—hypoglycemia—which causes severe metabolic changes that alter moods, thoughts, and behavior. Take a look at the list below, compiled by Mark Worden, from his 1980 article in the *Journal of Orthomolecular Medicine*. It compares commonly reported dry-drunk symptoms to those known to be caused by hypoglycemia.

Dry-Drunk Syndrome	Hypoglycemia
Irritability	Irritability
Depression	Depression
Aggressiveness	Aggressiveness
Insomnia	Insomnia
Fatigue	Fatigue
Restlessness	Restlessness
Confusion	Confusion
Desire to drink	Desire to drink
Nervousness	Nervousness

Typically, most of these symptoms occur in newly abstinent alcoholics who try to overcome their emotional and physical discomfort by smoking cigarettes excessively and drinking enormous amounts of coffee laced with sugar. Their pockets are stuffed with candy bars, and they habitually reach for colas for a quick lift. Their diets often consist of junk food high in refined sugars and low in quality protein, vegetables, grains, and fruits.

Both caffeine and nicotine cured with corn, beet, and cane sugars can prompt the outpouring of adrenaline that temporarily raises blood sugar, as do candies, baked goods, and other foods containing refined sugars. The relief provided by these quick fixes is short-lived. A surge of insulin quickly pushes glucose levels back below normal, and the symptoms and the need for a sugar fix begin all over again.

Maintaining constant and adequate glucose levels is one of our most important biochemical needs. Continued blood-sugar fluctuations to below amounts needed by the brain for stable functioning are a more logical explanation of dry-drunk symptoms than any psychological concept can be.

Controlling Hypoglycemia

You cannot recover from hypoglycemia overnight, but in a few short weeks you can feel much better. You can banish symptoms and correct the underlying metabolic errors just as our HRC clients do by following a healthy new diet and taking some more nutritional supplements. You'll have to give up both caffeine and cigarettes, but the sacrifice will pay enormous dividends in renewed energy and vibrant good health.

The Diet

Get ready for a big change in the way you eat. You're going to have to give up foods containing refined sugar. That means virtually all sweets. Candy bars. Colas. Cookies. Ice cream. I know you love these foods. You may not want them when you're drinking, but most alcoholics begin to crave sweets as soon as they go on the wagon. Small wonder! Did you ever think about the similarities between sugar and alcohol? Both are carbohydrates with no nutritional value—all you get from them is calories. Both are absorbed directly into the bloodstream, and both can cause memory blackouts and intense cravings. I can't promise you that giving up sugar will be easy. But with the nutritional support you'll get while you're on the diet, it won't be as bad as you think.

In addition to sugars, the diet also temporarily eliminates dairy products and wheat. Both are highly allergenic, and one or both frequently contribute to problems of alcohol allergy/addiction. You'll know within two weeks whether or not you are affected. If not, you can resume eating dairy products and foods containing wheat.

You will find the diet at the end of this chapter. There are lists of foods you can eat and those you must avoid. I've also provided suggested menus and meal preparation and shopping tips. Don't let the word "diet" scare you. You are not about to embark on a regime of grapefruit and lettuce leaves. You will be pleasantly surprised by the enormous variety of foods you can choose from. You will be eating three hearty meals each day, plus healthy and filling midmorning, midafternoon, and after-dinner snacks. In fact, you probably will be eating more and better than you have in years.

It is important to eat all the snacks. They will provide you with a steady supply of protein, fats, and slowly available (complex) carbohydrates to prevent the drop in blood sugar that normally occurs about two hours after a meal. If your meals are delayed for any reason, you may need an extra snack.

Key Nutrients That Block Sugar Cravings

Your cravings for sweets could sabotage all your efforts. But you can combat them with—you guessed it—many of the nutrients you are already taking, plus two new ones. Your old friends glutamine, vitamin C, magnesium, and pantothenic acid help keep sugar cravings under control. Two others, niacin and chromium, will heighten this effect. Add two 500-mg doses of niacin, one at breakfast, one at supper; you are already getting enough chromium in your multivitamin formula.

Both niacin and chromium have proved extremely helpful in the treatment of alcoholism. Let's take a look at what they can do.

Niacin

In his second communication to AA physicians, Bill Wilson reported that about 70 percent of alcoholics who took niacin (vitamin B_3) found that they felt much better: "Evidence has mounted that many of this group reporting recoveries from depression, anxiety, tension, etc., are actually hypoglycemics, people in whom B_3 is, to a considerable degree, preventing the abnormal drop of blood sugar which is characteristic of that malady."

Wilson quotes several physicians who were treating alcoholics with niacin. One of these doctors, Jack Ward, M.D., a psychiatrist in Trenton, New Jersey, speculated that "the good response of the 'unhappy sobriety types' to niacin . . . is due at least in part to the effect of the B_3 on the blood-sugar levels."

Wilson also reported on the work of Russell Smith, M.D., nephew of AA cofounder Dr. Bob Smith. Russell Smith treated 507 hard-core alcoholics with six grams of niacin a day for six months. He found that 340 did very well indeed. They remained sober and their memories improved, as did their learning abilities, problem-solving skills, coping abilities, sleep, appetites, interpersonal relationships, and job performance. Another 98 reported improvements in well-being and energy. Their moods were also more stable. Of the 507, only 66 did not respond positively to the niacin therapy.

Niacin is remarkably safe even when taken without medical supervision. There has never been a reported overdose death. However, bear in mind the following precautions:

- Since high doses can affect the liver, *do not* take niacin if your lab tests reveal any abnormalities of liver function. You can begin after you correct your liver problems.
- Niacin may cause flushing due to the sudden release of histamine it triggers. You don't have to give up taking niacin. The redness and itching is not harmful and will eventually disappear.
- A dose that is too high for you can cause nausea and vomiting

after a few days. This gastric distress disappears twenty-four to forty-eight hours after discontinuing niacin.

- Niacin may elevate blood sugar in some diabetics. If so, substitute niacinamide, another form of Vitamin B_3; it will have no effect on insulin requirements.

Chromium

This mineral is essential for sugar metabolism. Refined sugars force a 20 percent increase in the excretion of chromium into the blood, depleting the stores needed to control abnormal glucose fluctuations.

Take chromium picolinate, not inorganic chromium salts. Chromium picolinate is the newest and best absorbed kind of chromium. It will help stabilize blood sugar by raising levels that are too low or lowering levels that are too high.

Chromium levels were extremely low in ninety-one of the one hundred alcoholics participating in our HRC study. (The only client with high chromium levels had been wearing a chromium wire brace in his mouth. Alcohol eroded the metal, causing him to ingest chromium particles, which were then stored in his tissues.) Chromium picolinate will speed improvement in glucose availability and reverse your hypoglycemic symptoms.

Incidentally, you may be interested to know that chromium can protect you against stroke and heart attack. In countries where chromium intake and tissue levels are high, the incidence of heart attack and stroke is low. What's more, tests of patients with severe heart disease have shown that they have virtually no chromium available in the aorta, the heart's major artery. There is also good medical evidence that chromium deficiency contributes to the buildup of plaque, the fatty deposits that clog coronary arteries and precipitate heart attacks.

Other Important Nutrients

You learned about glutamine, vitamin C, magnesium, and pantothenic acid in Chapter 6, but you may be interested to know how they help control hypoglycemia and stave off cravings for sugar.

Glutamine:

In the brain, glutamine is converted to glutamic acid, the only alternate source of glucose available to the brain. It provides a ready source of brain fuel for hypoglycemics and helps stave off sugar cravings and hypoglycemic symptoms that develop when blood-sugar levels drop too low.

Vitamin C:

Vitamin C is very effective against stress. The adrenal glands use large amounts for hormone production. Adrenal supplies of vitamin C can become severely depleted as a result of hypoglycemia and associated sugar cravings.

Magnesium:

Supplements help to stabilize blood-sugar levels of hypoglycemics.

Pantothenic Acid:

Alcohol destroys the pantothenic acid needed for normal production of all the adrenal hormones, including cortisone. Under these circumstances, the adrenal glands lose their ability to protect you from stress. As you now know, hypoglycemia also weakens the adrenals. Replacing lost pantothenic acid will help repair the damage.

Caffeine and Nicotine Have to Go

Before you close this book and say, "That's it! I can't follow this @##%% program!" let me assure you that I do not expect you to stop smoking cigarettes and drinking coffee right now. But both will have to go in the near future.

As you know, caffeine and nicotine aggravate hypoglycemia by setting in motion that now-familiar scenario in which the adrenals release adrenaline in response to low blood sugar, prompting the liver to release glycogen. Blood sugar then rises, and the pancreas begins to pump out insulin, overshooting the mark and causing another drop in blood sugar. The result is a quick, short-lived lift followed by fatigue that can last for hours. If you continue to drink coffee and smoke, your body will pay a high price. Every one of our follow-up studies shows that the 20 to 25 percent of HRC clients who relapsed were those who could not (or would not) stop smoking cigarettes.

Caffeine

There is no question that caffeine can wire you and bring on restlessness, depression, irritability, anxiety, insomnia, shakiness, and bone-tired fatigue. Consider the case of Brent, a young waiter admitted to our clinic last year. He was subject to sudden panic attacks, spells of heart pounding and overpowering fearfulness that his physician had been treating with the drug Inderal, a blood-pressure medication that has a calming effect. After we convinced Brent to give up the forty cups of coffee he had been drinking daily, his panic attacks, as well as his insomnia and tremors, disappeared.

If you are drinking five or more cups of coffee a day, you may develop severe headaches, listlessness, and nervousness if you stop cold turkey. You will do better by reducing your daily intake gradually over the course of a week. Do not substitute decaffeinated coffee. Instead, switch to caffeine-free herbal teas or sparkling water with lime or lemon.

You will soon be rewarded for all these sacrifices with more energy, more restful sleep, and, most important, reduced cravings for sugar and alcohol.

Nicotine Addiction

Almost every smoker admitted to HRC wants to quit smoking but can't. That isn't surprising. Nicotine is probably the most addictive substance known. Let me tell you about John, a client who came to us after his release from a detox center. He had been in detox almost every weekend that year. Although he was only twenty-eight, he had been in four treatment programs. None had worked for him.

In the middle of our initial interview, John stood up and announced that he had to smoke a cigarette. He told me he smoked two and a half packs a day but wished he could quit. I suggested that by detoxifying his brain and body systems, his cravings for alcohol would disappear. Although he was miserably ill with alcoholism, he had a bright, inquiring mind. He agreed to follow our biochemical repair program to the letter to see if I was right.

Giving up cigarettes was almost harder for John than giving up alcohol. With the help of a prescription for Nicorette gum and the very same nutrient program I am recommending to you, he went off to the north woods of Minnesota for a weekend and came back a nonsmoker. It has been almost a year since he completed treatment. He has remained free of all drugs and continues to maintain his healthy new life-style.

Millions of people have successfully quit smoking. With the proper tools and support, you will too.

But don't worry. I'm not going to ask you to quit smoking . . . yet. Instead, concentrate on staying free of alcohol, refined sugars, and caffeine. After you rid your system of these toxic substances, your body will be much more cooperative when you stop smoking. For the time being, just be aware of how many cigarettes you smoke every day and try to cut down a little.

Now, let's take a look at the diet you will be using to bring hypoglycemic symptoms under control.

The HRC Hypoglycemic (Antiallergy) Diet for Alcoholics

This diet is extremely healthy. It is high in complex carbohydrates and, as I explained earlier, temporarily eliminates dairy products and wheat. Before you begin, read the following instructions:

- One meal each day should consist largely of vegetables. Big salads will do the trick.
- When buying food, read labels carefully. Most canned soup and juice, ketchup, mayonnaise, mustard, salad dressing, and canned vegetables contain sugar and/or starch. You can get sugar-free products at food co-ops or health-food stores.

- *Do not* use any food that lists sugar among the first four ingredients on the label.
- Throw out junk food containing refined sugar. You will be snacking on healthy foods frequently so you won't feel hungry.
- Substitute soy milk or fresh goat's milk or Rice Dream (Imagine Foods, Palo Alto, California) for cow's milk. Some HRC clients are afraid that goat's milk will taste terrible, but most find that it tastes just like cow's milk (but, I admit, it depends on the goat).
- Avoid aspirin compounds including Anacin; Empirin, cold tablets; Midol, Trigesic, and medications containing alcohol (read the labels). Bayer aspirin is caffeine free and may be used.

Suggested Daily Menus

Here are a few samples of the kind of healthy meals you can choose. Remember, one meal each day should consist largely of vegetables.

Breakfast:
Two eggs (cooked any style)
One slice bread (millet or brown rice)
A beverage from the list on page 136
Fresh fruit in season
A handful of raw almonds, sesame seeds, or pumpkin seeds

or

One cup cooked cereal: millet, buckwheat, or oats with goat's milk or soy milk

Midmorning snack:
Five to ten raw almonds or other raw, unroasted nuts

or

One piece of fresh fruit: pear, pineapple, papaya, melon, or a bowl of cherries

or

One slice toasted rice or millet bread with almond or sunflower butter

or

½ large or one small avocado

or

Tomato or V-8 juice (12 oz)

or

Orange or grapefruit juice diluted with spring water (two parts
water to one part juice)

or

One slice whole-grain bread (other than wheat)
One pat margarine (other than corn-oil type)

or

Beans and brown rice with fresh tomato, onion, garlic

or

½ cup drained canned salmon, tuna, or sardines
Small vegetable salad

or

Any breakfast choice

Lunch:
Hamburger patty
Tossed salad with natural dressing (dairy free) or avocado with
mushrooms sautéed in olive oil
Fresh peach
Acceptable beverage

or

Large bowl of freshly prepared vegetable, mushroom, pea, or lentil
soup (not creamed)
Fresh fruit in season

or

Broiled fish
Cooked or steamed vegetable such as green beans, carrots, broccoli, cauliflower, zucchini

Midafternoon snack:
Same choices as midmorning snack

Dinner:
Broiled chicken (remove skin)
½ baked potato
Green or wax beans
One slice whole-grain bread (other than wheat) with almond, cashew, or sunflower butter
Mixed raw vegetables
Strawberries (10–12)
Acceptable beverage

After-dinner snack:
Same choices as midmorning snack

Unless otherwise noted, all foods are measured raw.

Foods to Avoid

Beverages

Alcoholic beverages

Cocoa

Coffee

Decaffeinated coffee

Colas

Ovaltine

Soft drinks*

Diet soft drinks

Strong tea

Desserts

Cake

Chocolate

Cookies

Custard

Dessert topping

Ice cream

Jell-O

Pastry

Pie

Pudding

Fruits

Dried fruits (including raisins)

*Exceptions include club soda, seltzer, and natural sparkling waters like Perrier.

Fruits canned in syrup
Grapes

Grains
Dry, sweetened cereal
Crackers (white)
Grits
Matzo
Pancakes/waffles
Pizza
Pretzels
Rolls
White rice
White, whole wheat bread
Avoid white flour in any form;
whole grains, other than wheat
flour, may be used

Meats
Canned meats
Cold cuts
Hot dogs
Salami
Sausage
Bacon

Sweets
Artificial sweeteners
Candy
Caramel
Chewing gum
Honey
Jam/jelly
Malt
Marmalade
Molasses
Sugar (refined, corn, beet)
Maple syrup
Other forms of sugar: dextrose,
fructose, glucose, hexitol,
lactose, maltose, mannitol,
sorbitol, sucrose

Vegetables
Corn chips
French fries
Potato chips
Sweet pickles
Sweet relishes

Allowable Foods

Beverages
Apricot juice
Carrot juice
Clear broth
Herb teas
Lemon juice
Lime juice

Loganberry juice
Orange juice
Pineapple juice
Raspberry juice
Sauerkraut juice
Tangerine juice
V-8 juice

(Dilute all fruit juices, 2 parts
spring water to 1 part juice)

Fats
Salad oils

Fruit (fresh)
Apples
Apricots
Avocado
Blueberries
Cantaloupe
Casaba melon
Cherries
Coconut (fresh)
Fruit salad (without grapes)
Grapefruit
Honeydew melon
Lemon
Lime
Muskmelon
Oranges
Peaches
Pears
Pineapple
Plums
Raspberries
Rhubarb (no sugar added)
Strawberries
Tangerines

Nuts and Seeds
Almonds
Brazil nuts

Peanuts
Pecans
Pumpkin seeds
Sesame seeds
Sunflower seeds
Walnuts

Protein
Chicken and other fowl
Eggs
Fish
Meat (unprocessed)
Shellfish
Tofu (soy)

Sprouts
Alfalfa
Bean

Vegetables (fresh)
Artichokes (globe or French)
Asparagus
Beans (green or wax)
Beets
Broccoli
Cabbage
Cauliflower
Celery
Cucumbers
Lettuce
Mushrooms
Olives
Onions (green or raw)
Parsley

Peas (green or edible pod)
Peppers
Pickles (dill or sour)
Pimentos
Radishes
Rutabaga
Sauerkraut
Soybeans
Spinach
Squash (Hubbard or winter)

Tomatoes
Water chestnuts
Zucchini

Whole grains
Barley
Buckwheat
Millet
Oats
Rice (brown or wild)

Shopping Tips

- Choose foods that are as close to their natural state as possible: fresh vegetables and fruits; fresh meats, fish, chicken, and eggs; raw nuts and seeds; and fresh salad greens.
- Avoid canned, processed, dyed, chemically flavored, frozen, additive-laden foods.
- If you can't find millet bread or brown rice bread at your supermarket, try a food cooperative. Some health-food stores also carry these whole-grain substitutes for wheat bread. Before you buy rye or oat bread, read the label. Wheat is usually the first ingredient listed.
- Don't buy roasted nuts. The process of high-heat roasting causes undesirable changes in the natural oils the nuts contain. In the body, this altered oil can promote formation of free radicals, dangerously unstable molecules capable of damaging healthy tissue and promoting the development of cancer. Choose only raw nuts and seeds.
- Pass up luncheon meats (Spam, bacon, ham, bologna). They are loaded with refined sugars and cancer-causing nitrates.
- You can find fruit-sweetened jams at a food co-op or health-food store.
- Drink flavored sparkling water (read the label to confirm that it is sugar free).

- Cut your salt intake by using lite salt, which is half potassium (needed for cellular energy) and half sodium.

Meal Preparation Tips

- Peel fruits and vegetables or remove outer layers to avoid pesticide residues.
- Steam your vegetables (if you cook them in water, you will lose much of their vitamin and mineral content). You can get a steamer that fits inside any pot in most housewares departments. Cook vegetables until they are almost tender, not soggy.
- Raw vegetables are your best choice; they also make excellent snacks.
- Use fruit juice on cereal if you don't have soy, rice, or goat's milk. (The ban on cow's milk is only a temporary measure until you have had your allergy test.)
- Keep a lot of assorted nuts, sunflower seeds, apples, oranges, carrot sticks, celery, and other raw vegetables on hand for snacking.

Getting Well and Getting Better

So there you have it—the program you will use to recover your health. You may be surprised to learn that we already have covered all the common ground there is among alcoholics. From here on in, you can pick and choose the treatments that suit you best. In the next chapter we will review the results of your lab tests so that you can begin to repair any damage they reveal. After that, you can zero in on your individual problems. You will find nutrient formulas to help you overcome the common symptoms related to alcoholism.

When we get to this point in the program, HRC clients often announce that they have turned into health nuts. And when we ask about cravings, they are inclined to quip that they are too busy taking pills and planning meals to think about drinking! Humor aside, they have witnessed the amazing power of the nutritional supplements to restore their energy, clarity of mind, and sense of well-being. I fully expect you will as well.

Eight

Week Four:
Tailoring Repair

If you have not yet begun to feel better, this is the week that will prove to you that this program really works. Although I still worry about clients who don't begin to improve early on, I have learned to be patient. Experience has taught me that Week Four can make all the difference. I had to remind myself of this last winter when we had two severely depressed women in the program. During their first three weeks, Anita and Mary Jo sat glum and listless while the others slowly perked up. Reviewing their records, I saw that since childhood, both women had exhibited a pattern of depression that can require taking large doses of Efamol for a while before the bleak moods are eliminated. Sure enough, for both women Week Four was a turning point. Suddenly they were laughing and chatting happily.

Some clients feel so good by this point that they don't think they need anything else. What about you? Even if you're feeling better than you have in years, ask yourself if any of your medical tests have indicated liver abnormalities, thyroid disorders, or potentially harmful accumulations of toxic metals. Perhaps you've been having trouble sleeping. Or you may be tired too much of the time. What about pain? Or shakiness? There is no reason to tolerate any of these symptoms. You can overcome them with the aid of the nutrient formulas on the pages ahead.

Ask yourself too about psychological symptoms—anxiety, paranoia, obsessive-compulsive behavior, chronic stress, or memory problems—all common complaints among recovering alcoholics. Many of these symptoms are directly related to the biochemistry of the brain; some are the results of depletion of minerals our bodies need for good health. All can be eliminated by resupplying the nutrients needed to normalize and stabilize your emotions.

Now's the time for you to begin using the nutrient replacement lists (Charts 6 and 7) that will help you keep track of the nutrients you're taking on your adjusted nutrient plan. In the weeks ahead, you will probably be adding even more nutrients to those you are taking now. If you follow these simple instructions, you will have no trouble keeping track of what you take:

1. To add a nutrient, find it on your nutrient replacement list. If it is not there, enter it in the blank space provided at the end of the list.

2. If you already are taking a nutrient called for in one of the formulas, increase the amount you presently take to the level of the new formula. *Do not* add the full formula dose to what you already are taking. Here is an example:

   Your multivitamin/mineral formula includes a daily dose of 600 milligrams of vitamin B_5 (pantothenic acid). The antistress formula in this chapter calls for 1,000 milligrams of B_5 daily. All you have to do is add 400 milligrams $(1,000 - 600)$ to the amount you already take and enter the new total in the column headed Combination Total. You may have to round out the milligrams to the nearest 25 or 50. A few extra won't hurt.

3. If a formula calls for the same dose of a nutrient you already take, *do not* double the amount. Your current dose will serve the purpose.

Chart 6. Nutrient Replacement List for II ADH/THIQ and Omega-6 EFA Deficient Alcoholics

Combination Total	Nutrient	Number of Capsules	Daily Dose
	Glutamine (500 mg)	6	3,000 mg
	Free-form amino acids (750 mg)	6	4,500 mg
	DL-Phenylalanine (500 mg)	3	1,500 mg
	Tryptophan* (500 mg)	2–4	1,000–2,000 mg
	Vitamin C (ascorbic acid) (1,000 mg)	6	6,000 mg
	Calcium/magnesium (300/150 mg)	4	1,200/600 mg
	Efamol (500 mg)	6	3,000 mg
	Pancreatic enzymes (425 mg)	6	2,550 mg
	Multivitamin/mineral	6	
	Vitamin A (palmitate)		24,000 IU
	Vitamin B_1 (thiamine)		120 mg
	Vitamin B_2 (riboflavin)		60 mg
	Vitamin B_3 (niacinamide)		180 mg
	Vitamin B_5 (pantothenic acid)		600 mg
	Vitamin B_6 (pyridoxine)		180 mg
	Pyridoxal-5^1-phosphate		6 mg
	Vitamin B_{12} (cobalamine)		480 mcg
	Folic acid		360 mcg
	Biotin		480 mcg
	PABA		240 mg
	Vitamin E		480 IU
1,100 mg	Calcium		300 mg

Header over the Combination Total / Nutrient columns: **Daily Intake (from Adjusted Nutrient Plan)**

Chart 6. Nutrient Replacement List for II ADH/THIQ and Omega-6 EFA Deficient Alcoholics (Continued)

Daily Intake (from Adjusted Nutrient Plan)			
Combination Total	Nutrient	Number of Capsules	Daily Dose
900 mg	Magnesium		300 mg
	Potassium		120 mg
	Manganese		18 mg
	Zinc		36 mg
	Copper		1.8 mg
	Selenium		240 mcg
	Vanadium		240 mcg
	Molybdenum		240 mcg
	Glutamic acid		240 mg
	Chromium		480 mcg
	Iron		24 mg
	Antioxidant complex	1	
44,000 IU	Vitamin A (beta-carotene)		20,000 IU
	Glutathione		60 mg
	Methionine		40 mg
630 IU	Vitamin E		150 IU
	Dimethylglycine		80 mg
	Cysteine		80 mg
3,040 mg	Vitamin C		40 mg
46 mg	Zinc		10 mg
270 mcg	Selenium		30 mcg
	Ubiquinone		500 mcg
	Lipoic acid		2.5 mg
	Omega-3 EFA (fortified flax)	2 Tbsp	4,600 mg
1,180 mg	Niacin (500 mg)	2	1,000 mg

Add formulas you want to use as you find them in the following chapters. Keep a running total of combined nutrient amounts in the left-hand column.
*Use only if the FDA lifts the current ban on its sale.

Chart 7. Nutrient Replacement List for Allergic/Addicted Alcoholics

Daily Intake (from Adjusted Nutrient Plan)			
Combination Total	Nutrient	Number of Capsules	Daily Dose
	Glutamine (500 mg)	6	3,000 mg
	Free-form amino acids (750 mg)	4	3,000 mg
	DL-Phenylalanine (500 mg)	2	1,000 mg
	Tryptophan* (500 mg)	2–4	1,000–2,000 mg
	Vitamin C (ascorbic acid) (1,000 mg)	4	4,000 mg
	Calcium/magnesium (300/150 mg)	4	1,200/600 mg
	Efamol (500 mg)	4	2,000 mg
	Pancreatic enzymes (425 mg)	6	2,550 mg
	Multivitamin/mineral	6	
	Vitamin A (palmitate)		24,000 IU
	Vitamin B_1 (thiamine)		120 mg
	Vitamin B_2 (riboflavin)		60 mg
	Vitamin B_3 (niacinamide)		180 mg
	Vitamin B_5 (pantothenic acid)		600 mg
	Vitamin B_6 (pyridoxine)		180 mg
	Pyridoxal-5'-phosphate		6 mg
	Vitamin B_{12} (cobalamine)		480 mcg
	Folic acid		360 mcg
	Biotin		480 mcg
	PABA		240 mg
	Vitamin E		480 IU
1,100 mg	Calcium		300 mg

Chart 7. Nutrient Replacement List for
Allergic/Addicted Alcoholics *(Continued)*

Daily Intake (from Adjusted Nutrient Plan)			
Combination Total	**Nutrient**	**Number of Capsules**	**Daily Dose**
900 mg	Magnesium		300 mg
	Potassium		120 mg
	Manganese		18 mg
	Zinc		36 mg
	Copper		1.8 mg
	Selenium		240 mcg
	Vanadium		240 mcg
	Molybdenum		240 mcg
	Glutamic acid		240 mcg
	Chromium		480 mcg
	Iron		21.6 mg
	Antioxidant complex	1	
44,000 IU	Vitamin A (beta-carotene)		20,000 IU
	Glutathione		60 mg
	Methionine		40 mg
630 IU	Vitamin E		150 IU
	Dimethylglycine		80 mg
	Cysteine		80 mg
4,040 mg	Vitamin C		40 mg
46 mg	Zinc		10 mg
270 mcg	Selenium		30 mcg
	Ubiquinone		500 mcg
	Lipoic acid		2.5 mg
	Omega-3 EFA (fortified flax)	2 Tbsp	4,600 mg
1,180 mg	Niacin or niacinamide	2 (500 mg)	1,000 mg

Add formulas you want to use as you find them in the following chapters. Keep a running total of combined nutrient amounts in the left-hand column.
*Add only if the FDA lifts the current ban on its sale.

As you read the sections ahead, you will see that the same symptoms can be caused by shortages of a number of different nutrients. For example, not getting enough B-complex vitamins can cause depression, fatigue, and anxiety. There is no way to determine exactly what deficiency is to blame for any of your symptoms; my advice is to take adequate amounts of the nutrients in every formula you feel you need.

Each formula in this chapter comes with instructions that tell you whether to add more of a given nutrient to the amounts you are taking or whether you already are taking enough. If you follow instructions, you will be in no danger of overdosing. (You can refer to Tables 23 and 24 in Chapter 9 for maximum safe doses of each nutrient.)

You may be dismayed at the thought of taking even more nutrients. Often, all you will have to do is increase your dosage slightly. Swallowing a few more capsules is a small price to pay for the physical and emotional equilibrium you will achieve when you complete this program. Certainly your health is worth the inconvenience.

To determine what new nutrients you'll need to achieve better physical health, we first need to review the results of the medical tests we have not yet addressed: your liver function, thyroid, serum zinc, serum histamine, and hair analysis. We'll consider the nutrients that can help you overcome the problems revealed by these tests. Then we'll discuss the chemically induced emotional problems that so often sabotage recovery from alcoholism, and the ways you can treat them through nutritional therapy.

Continuing Physical Repair

Liver Function

If any of your lab tests suggest that your liver is not functioning properly, your physician undoubtedly has urged you to stop drinking. You can do much more than that. You can actually help to repair the liver damage alcohol has inflicted. At HRC we have learned that a combination of two amino acids—carnitine and methionine—the vitamins choline and inositol, plus Efamol and a remarkable substance called silymarin help to restore normal liver function (Table 9). Each nutrient has a specific role in this repair process:

- *Carnitine* helps the liver oxidize the heavy fatty-acid load produced by drinking.
- Substances called *lipotropic factors,* which contain methionine, choline, and inositol, can rid the liver of the fat accumulated during years of alcohol abuse. (Healthy liver cells can regenerate indefinitely, but with continued alcohol abuse, cells fill with fat and die.) At HRC we use LIPO-3 Factors formulated by Richlife, Costa Mesa, California.
- *Efamol,* as you know from earlier chapters, contains gamma-linolenic acid (GLA), which can prevent liver damage. At HRC we use Efamol from Murdock Pharmaceuticals, Springville, Utah.
- *Silymarin,* a nutrient I haven't mentioned before, has an astounding effect on the liver. This substance, also known as milk thistle extract, speeds liver regeneration. Studies with patients who have liver disease have shown that elevated liver readings

Table 9. The HRC Formula for Liver Repair		
Nutrient	**Dose**	**Directions**
Carnitine	500 mg	1 capsule 3 times per day
Lipotropic Factors:		1 capsule 3 times per day
Methionine*	100 mg	
Inositol	333 mg	
Choline	333 mg	
Efamol*	500 mg	6 capsules per day
Silymarin	50 mg	1 capsule 3 times per day

*This level was partly or completely established in your adjusted nutrient plan or in other formulas you may be taking. Refer to your nutrient replacement list (Chart 6 or 7) to determine whether you need to add more of this nutrient to achieve the level suggested here.

decreased significantly only among those treated with silymarin. And a study of patients with alcoholic cirrhosis of the liver found a significantly higher survival rate among those receiving silymarin. In addition, silymarin acts as a free radical scavenger in the liver—it attacks and destroys harmful free radical molecules that can induce disease and promote aging. You can get silymarin from Twin Laboratories, Ronkonkoma, New York.

Thyroid

The thyroid gland at the base of the neck stores and discharges thyroid hormones into the bloodstream. The most common thyroid disorder among alcoholics is hypothyroidism, or low thyroid function. Symptoms include fatigue, slow thinking, depression, hoarseness, dry and flaking skin, cold feet and hands, coarse or brittle hair, fingernails that are ridged and break easily, and sexual problems. There are several tests to measure specific thyroid hormones and a thyroid stimulation test to determine if thyroid function is normal. At HRC, results of these lab tests sometimes are within normal ranges, but a newer test, the fluorescence activated microsphere assay (FAMA), can reveal abnormalities the other procedures often miss. It can identify hypothyroid conditions that had been previously undetected, as well as disorders in which the body attacks the thyroid. If you have a thyroid disorder, you will require medication prescribed by your physician.

Serum Zinc

Chronic alcohol consumption and high sugar intake often force excess zinc excretion, which can lead to a deficiency. This in turn can permit copper levels to rise dangerously, which can bring on psychological disorders, including paranoia.

If your lab tests reveal that you are low on zinc but your copper levels are not elevated and you are not subject to paranoia, you can bring your zinc levels back to normal by taking twenty milligrams of zinc (one tablet) per day. For most efficient absorption, take your zinc on an empty stomach.

If your zinc is low and serum copper is high (this may also show up in your hair analysis results) and you *are* subject to paranoia, you can correct matters with our HRC formula for paranoia in Table 10. You can lower excess copper levels by taking zinc, which will gradually remove copper from your body tissues. Vitamin C and niacin are also powerful antidotes to excess copper. Interestingly, the estrogen in birth-control pills can raise copper levels and destroy zinc, so if you are on the pill you might want to consider another means of contraception.

Paranoia can also occur with low levels of histamine and folic acid and/or ongoing insomnia. Whatever, the underlying biochemical cause, paranoia is common among alcoholics. Therapy will not help.

Table 10. The HRC Formula for Paranoia

Nutrient	Dose	Directions
L-Tryptophan*†	500 mg	3 to 6 capsules as needed at bedtime
Zinc picolinate*	20 mg	1 capsule at breakfast; 1 at dinner
Vitamin C*	1,000 mg	1 capsule 3 times per day with meals
Niacin* (non-time released)	500 mg	1 capsule 2 times per day with meals
Folic acid*	800 mcg	1 capsule 3 times per day with meals
Vitamin B_{12}*	1,000 mcg (B_{12} is bottled in mcgs)	1 capsule per day or weekly by injection
Manganese gluconate*	10 mg	1 capsule at breakfast; 1 at dinner

*This level was partly or completely established in your adjusted nutrient plan or in other formulas you may be taking. Refer to your nutrient replacement list (Chart 6 or 7) to determine whether you need to add more of this nutrient to achieve the level suggested here.
†Use tryptophan only if the FDA lifts the current ban on its sale.

A few years ago I was horrified to read in *Newsweek* an account of how clients at a well-known treatment center were "helped" to overcome their paranoia. Their therapy required them to be blindfolded and spend many hours trusting others to help them find their way around!

Serum Histamine

Histamine is a major brain neurotransmitter and a brain-chemical modulator. If your lab tests show that your histamine levels are low, it is important to have your blood levels of copper measured (your hair analysis will give you some indication of your copper status). Copper destroys histamine in the brain. This process can cause violent behavior and depression as well as paranoia.

Low Histamine:

The alcohol biotype most likely to fit the profile of low histamine is the allergic/addicted alcoholic. If your histamine levels are low, you will need the HRC paranoia formula in Table 10 to restore these levels to the normal range. Besides lowering copper levels, other benefits of raising histamine levels are increased energy and libido, and needing less sleep. It was developed by the late Carl Pfeiffer, M.D., Ph.D., a histamine researcher and founder of the famed Princeton BioCenter in Skillman, New Jersey.

High Histamine:

High histamine levels can be a problem, too. IIADH/THIQ alcoholics are most likely to be affected. They are compulsive, obsessive, driven, highly sexed individuals who need very little sleep. When depressed, they are subject to suicidal tendencies. Dr. Pfeiffer determined that histamine levels will decrease and symptoms lessen in response to daily doses of methionine, an amino acid that detoxifies histamine in the brain. Calcium taken morning and evening also lowers histamine. Both are included in the HRC formula for Compulsiveness/Obsessiveness (Table 11), which contains Pfeiffer's recommended treatment for high histamine levels.

If your histamine level is extremely high, your physician may pre-

Table 11. The HRC Formula for Compulsiveness/Obsessiveness

Nutrient	Dose	Directions
L-Methionine*	500 mg	2 capsules per day between meals
L-Tryptophan*†‡	500 mg	1 capsule 3 times per day
Vitamin B$_6$*‡	100 mg	1 capsule 3 times per day with meals
Niacin*‡	500 mg	1 capsule with food
Calcium*	200 mg × 6 1,200 mg total	2 capsules 3 times per day with meals
Vitamin C*	1,000 mg	1 capsule 2 times per day with meals

*This level was partly or completely established in your adjusted nutrient plan or in other formulas you may be taking. Refer to your nutrient replacement list (Chart 6 or 7) to determine whether you need to add more of this nutrient to achieve the level suggested here.
†Use tryptophan only if the FDA lifts the current ban on its sale.
‡**Warnings:** Take tryptophan only if your histamine level is *not* high. Take vitamin B$_6$ and niacin only if you take tryptophan. Do *not* take niacin if your histamine is high as it will increase even more!
Take L-methionine only if your histamine level is high.

scribe the drug Dilantin, which works rapidly to bring it back to normal.

The formula also contains tryptophan. A study by J. Yaryura-Tobias, M.D., established that tryptophan combined with niacin and vitamin B$_6$ stabilized compulsive/obsessive patients in six months by increasing the availability of serotonin, the brain's calming neurotransmitter.

What Hair Analysis Can Show

Hair analysis is a better indicator than blood tests of toxic-metal accumulation. Metals can remain stored in tissues even when they don't show up in the blood. Results of your hair analysis will come with a printout of your mineral and toxic-metal levels like the example in Figure 7. You must have these results interpreted by a physician or nutritionist trained to appreciate their implications. Certain high readings may indicate storage of the mineral in question in the hair and soft tissues and an unavailability in blood and bone. It could thus be misleading to accept all your readings at face value.

The lab will provide duplicates of your results and the computerized analysis. Ask your doctor for these copies for your records. Based on the results of your hair analysis, you may be able to relate previously unexplained symptoms to accumulations of toxic metals in your body. Here is a brief summary of symptoms and treatment:

Cadmium

Cigarette paper contains cadmium and smokers inhale fumes from this metal with every cigarette. One pack contains 23 micrograms of cadmium. Excess intake of this metal can contribute to chronic bronchitis and/or emphysema. There is also a direct correlation between high blood pressure and cadmium intake. You can remove cadmium from your tissues with daily doses of zinc (40 milligrams), selenium (200 micrograms), and calcium (1,200 milligrams).

Mercury

Sugar-loving alcoholics tend to have terrible teeth with lots of mercury fillings. Recent reports about the effects of the mercury contained in these fillings help explain why so many also complain about aches and pains, depression, and fatigue. Some HRC clients have improved dramatically after their mercury fillings are removed. We then treat them with intravenous infusions of vitamin C to counteract the mercury their tissues have absorbed. Mercury poisoning can cause suicidal depression, fatigue, memory loss, headache, vision loss, speech disorders, emotional instability, and confusion. (The expression "mad as a hatter" comes from the days when mercury vapor was used to clean hats. The cleaners, then called hatters, became "mad" as a result of their mercury exposure.)

In some cases, mercury poisoning must be treated with EDTA

Figure 7. Sample Hair Analysis Report
Hair Element Analysis

NAME			
AGE	52	SEX	M
HAIR LOCATION	Head Hair		
SPECIMEN NUMBER	000000000		
DATE REC'D	04/10/90	DATE COMP'L.	04/10/90

Clinically Significant Hair Elements

Essential Elements	Hair Value (ppm)	Reference Range (ppm)	Suspicious (Below Reference Range)	Reference Range	Suspicious (Above Reference Range)
Calcium	203	200–600	*****************		
Magnesium	18.9	25–75	************		
Zinc	134	160–240	*************		
Copper	9.9	12–35	*************		
Chromium 《	0.15	0.5–1.5	*		

Toxic Elements	Hair Value (ppm)	Reference Range (ppm)	Low	Medium	High
Lead	3.94	< 20.0	***		
Mercury 《	0.40	< 2.5	*		
Cadmium	0.61	< 1.0	*********		
Arsenic 《	1.00	< 2.0	*		
Nickel	0.32	< 1.0	***		

Suggested Clinical Significance in Hair

Element	Hair Value (ppm)	Reference Range (ppm)	Below Reference Range	Reference Range	Above Reference Range
Sodium	35	150–200	****		
Potassium	20.8	75–180	*****		
Selenium 《	1.0	3–6	*		
Manganese	0.39	1.0–10.0	******		
Aluminum	8.35	< 20.0	*******		

Unknown Clinical Significance in Hair

Element	Hair Value (ppm)	Reference Range (ppm)	Below Reference Range	Reference Range	Above Reference Range
Cobalt 《	0.10	0.2–1.0	*		
Iron	24.1	20–50	**********************		
Lithium	0.07	0.1–0.8	********		
Molybdenum 《	0.10	0.1–1.0	*		
Phosphorus	143	100–170	*********************************		
Vanadium 《	0.04	0.5–1.0	*		

《 Indicates below detection limit; value given is detection limit.

< = less than   》 = less than   ppm = parts per million

chelation therapy. This involves intravenous administration of ethylenediaminetetraacetic acid, a substance that combines with metals like mercury, lead, and cadmium and removes them from the body. Your doctor will have to determine how many treatments you need. For a list of physicians who use EDTA chelation therapy, contact the American College of Advancement in Medicine, 23121 Verdugo Drive, Suite 204, Laguna Hills, CA 92653, (714) 583-7666.

Aluminum

Aluminum toxicity has been associated with both hyperactivity in children and with Alzheimer's disease. In early stages of aluminum absorption, before the "tangles" of nerve fibers characteristic of Alzheimer's disease appear, aluminum levels can be lowered with magnesium. Since you are already taking magnesium as part of your adjusted nutrient plan, all you have to do is increase your daily dosage to 1,200 milligrams. Adding one cup of Epsom salts to your bathwater can also help bring high aluminum levels back to normal.

Lead

Alcoholics who work as house painters, garage mechanics, or at other jobs that expose them to lead are at high risk of accumulating toxic levels of this mineral. Allergic/addicted alcoholics seem drawn to these jobs. A lead buildup can impair your concentration and shorten your attention span. Your thinking may also become muddled.

Megadoses of vitamin B_1 (200 milligrams daily) can help relieve these symptoms. Calcium (1,200 milligrams per day) also helps remove lead from the tissues. However, the preferred treatment for lead toxicity is EDTA chelation therapy combined with several injections of vitamin B_1.

Other Minerals

Your hair analysis will also determine your levels of calcium, magnesium, zinc, copper, and chromium. Elevated copper levels should be confirmed by a serum copper test. You will find a discussion of copper toxicity and its treatment earlier in this chapter in the section on zinc.

Allergy and Candida-Antibody Tests

There is so much to say about food allergies, chemical sensitivities, and candida-related complex that I am devoting an entire chapter to the subject. If any of your test results are positive, you will find the answers you seek in Chapter 11. If your test results are negative, you can skip that chapter; if you have not been tested, please read it very carefully. You may find an explanation for symptoms that have not responded to treatment.

The Chemistry of Emotions

The notion that nutritional deprivation can have devastating effects on behavior and emotions is not new. Some of the most compelling evidence was gathered in World War II in a study of a group of physically and psychologically healthy young conscientious objectors who volunteered for a six-month experiment in which their usual food intake was cut in half. All experienced dramatic psychological and physical changes that lingered long after the experiment ended and they resumed eating normally.

Some became so disturbed that they required hospitalization in a psychiatric ward. One became violent; another chopped off three of his fingers in response to the stress. Several feared that they were going crazy. Some wept a lot, talked of suicide, and displayed extraordinary emotional disturbances. Depression, anxiety, apathy, and extreme mood swings were common, as were frequent outbursts of irritability and anger.

The men stopped participating in group activities, became isolated, and expressed growing feelings of social inadequacy. They lost interest in sex and reported difficulties in concentrating and comprehending, even though IQ tests detected no change in their intellectual capacities. These emotional symptoms did not vanish after the study ended. Indeed, some of the men grew even more irritable, depressed, argumentative, and negative.

Alcoholics experience much the same semistarvation neurosis.

They develop "emotional" symptoms as a direct result of the unavailability of the brain and body chemicals needed for stable feelings, thoughts, and memory.

Until the last two decades, little was known about how brain chemicals influence emotions, behavior, and memory. We certainly had no idea how to resolve most chemically induced emotional problems. Even today, the formulas we use at HRC to help our clients overcome these problems are not widely available. They are on the frontier of scientific progress. As a rule, new research tends to lie dormant for a period before being universally applied. But why should you wait when these tools are available to you now? The first step is to understand and accept the concepts upon which this therapy is based.

Amino Acids and the Brain

Folklore has long held that the working of our brains is affected by what we put into our bodies. Today, scientific evidence supports this you-are-what-you-eat "mythology." We now know that the brain transmits messages and creates emotions by means of neurotransmitters. Proper functioning of these vital natural substances depends on an adequate supply of amino acids extracted from your diet.

If illness, drug use, or genetic predisposition destroys or prevents normal conversion of amino acids to neurotransmitters, behavior, moods, emotion, and memory will suffer. Heavy alcohol use can set these changes in motion long before it damages the liver or other organs. Its effects on brain chemistry can cause anxiety, depression, short attention span, hostile and aggressive behavior, poor memory, and drug and alcohol cravings.

Over time, heavy drinking brings about biochemical changes that block or destroy nutrients needed for normal neurotransmitter formation and function. Alcohol can also inflame the pancreas and damage liver cells, disrupting normal absorption of nutrients. The damage to the pancreas severely reduces the production and release of enzymes needed to digest protein. As a result, the process by which amino acids are extracted from protein cannot continue normally. With only a trickle of precursor amino acids available to the brain, neurotransmitter formation declines and the "emotional" symptoms develop. One recent study found low amino-acid availability among all of the chronic drug users tested.

You can see that the emotional problems stemming from these changes in brain chemistry cannot possibly be corrected with talk therapy. But in the past, that has been the only treatment available. The HRC program gives you a more rational alternative. Now that we understand the physical basis for these problems, we can correct them by restoring brain biochemistry to normal.

Amino-Acid Replacement

Let me reassure you once again that it is safe to take amino acids. They are food. They are nontoxic. If you do not need a particular amino acid—if your body already has an adequate supply—the excess will be processed and then excreted through the urine. The chance of high doses of one amino acid adversely affecting levels of others by creating deficiencies is remote. Dr. Eric Braverman, a prominent amino-acid researcher, tells us that blood levels of an amino acid can increase three-fold without affecting the concentration of any of the other amino acids.

However, as I explained in Chapter 6, some people should not take amino acids. For your convenience and to emphasize the importance of the precautions I want you to take, I am repeating the warnings here.

Do not take any form of phenylalanine (D or L) if any of the following applies to you:

- You have PKU (phenylketonuria, a genetic error in phenylalanine metabolism)
- You have hepatic cirrhosis (liver disease)

Do not take either form of phenylalanine or L-tyrosine or L-tryptophan if you are taking an MAO inhibitor like Nardil or Parnate. However, *with your doctor's approval,* you can substitute amino acids for MAO inhibitors.

Do not take histidine if you have a history of schizophrenia and your histamine levels are above the normal range. High histamine levels have been linked to a factor in one of the schizophrenias, called histadelia.

Do not take tyrosine, DL-phenylalanine, or L-phenylalanine if you have high blood pressure. You can take these amino acids after your pressure has been reduced and stabilized.

Do not take any amino acids except with the approval and supervision of your physician under the following circumstances:

- You have systemic lupus erythematosus
- You have an inborn error of amino-acid metabolism
- You are on methadone therapy

I want to reassure you that the medical advisor for this book and I have carefully reviewed the repair program. All the formulas have been used at HRC for up to ten years. None of our clients has developed any problems. However, we cannot overemphasize the importance of consulting a physician before beginning this or any other new health program. If any of these natural substances appear to worsen a condition, stop using it immediately and consult your doctor.

WARNING: *If you have been diagnosed as schizophrenic, if you have a genetic error in amino-acid metabolism, or if you take an MAO inhibitor, undertake this program only under the supervision of a physician.*

The Healing Powers of Amino Acids

Amino-acid therapy is a powerful natural means of healing and repair. These substances are safer than drugs and often produce the same results. Dr. Carl Pfeiffer, founder of the Princeton BioCenter and pioneer amino-acid researcher, offers us Pfeiffer's Law:

We have found that if a drug can be found to do the job of medical healing, a nutrient can be found to do the same job. For example, anti-depressants usually enhance the effect of serotonin or the epinephrines. We now know that if we give the amino acids tryptophan or tyrosine, the body will synthesize these neurotransmitters, thereby achieving the same effect . . . The challenge of the future is to replace (or sometimes combine) drugs with these natural healers.

At Health Recovery Center, we rely on amino acids rather than drugs to treat emotional problems. We know that amino acids are safe, and there is ample evidence that they are effective. Clearly, if they weren't safe, the U.S. Food and Drug Administration would not permit their sale without a physician's prescription. But I want you to feel thoroughly confident about using these natural chemicals. For that reason, I'll give you a crash course in amino acids to familiarize you with their functions in the body and their ability to normalize and stabilize your emotions.

The Biological Tasks of Amino Acids

In the body, amino acids

- Create body tissues and cells
- Promote growth and repair of all parts of the body
- Create the enzymes required for digestion and production of hormones
- Promote proper functioning of the blood
- Make possible the communication within the brain, and between the brain and the rest of the nervous system
- Create energy as they are converted to glucose, blood sugar, and glycogen (sugar stored by the liver for release to meet energy needs)

Use Table 12 as your guide to amino acids and what they can do for you.

Table 12. The Amino Acids: Our Natural Pharmacy

Alanine

Converts quickly to usable glucose and prolongs stabilization of blood sugar (helpful for hypoglycemics). Reduces elevated triglycerides in diabetics; may be helpful in preventing seizures.

Table 12. The Amino Acids:
Our Natural Pharmacy (*Continued*)

Arginine

Induces release of growth hormone from the pituitary; increases sperm count; detoxifies ammonia, which is helpful in cirrhosis of the liver; stimulates the immune response by enhancing production of T cells.

Warnings:

* *Use carefully in schizophrenic conditions*
* *May cause replication of herpes simplex virus; keep intake low in affected individuals*

Aspartic Acid (Asparagine)

Protects the liver; helps detoxify ammonia; promotes uptake of trace minerals in the intestinal tract.

Carnitine

Helps mobilize cellulite and other surface fats; helps combat fatigue and muscular weakness; helps provide energy for tissues by promoting oxidation of long-chain fatty acids; useful in clearing triglycerides from the blood.

Citrulline

A precursor of the amino acids arginine and ornithine; plays a role in the detoxification of ammonia; stimulates growth hormone.

Cysteine

Helps repair tissues damaged by alcohol abuse, cigarette smoke, and air pollution through detoxification of acetaldehyde; helps maintain skin flexibility and texture; promotes red- and white-blood-cell reproduction and tissue restoration in lung diseases; promotes iron absorption; helps prevent formation of harmful peroxidized fats and free radicals; protects the lungs against damage from cigarette smoke; used in treatment of bronchial disease and asthma.

Fhreomine

An immunostimulant that promotes thymus gland growth. Useful in treating spastic disorders. Deficiency, if severe, causes neurologic dysfunction.

GABA (Gamma-Aminobutyric Acid)

Useful in inducing calm and tranquility; may be useful in treatment of schizophrenia, epilepsy, depression, high blood pressure, high-stress disorders, manic behavior, and acute agitation.

Glutamic Acid

Precursor of GABA and glutamine. Taken by mouth, glutamic acid cannot cross the blood-brain barrier. Do not substitute for glutamine.

Glutamine

Antistress effect; useful in treatment of alcoholism by reducing cravings for alcohol and sugar. Improves memory and dexterity.

Glycine

Can be used as a beverage sweetener; decreases uric-acid levels to reverse gout; useful in epilepsy and other conditions characterized by abnormal nerve firings.

Histidine

Creates an antianxiety effect in the brain; promotes good hearing by stimulating auditory nerves; a promising answer for rhumatoid arthritis, releases histamines from body stores for sexual arousal.
Warnings:

- *Use carefully in manic-depressive patients with elevated histamine levels*
- *Take with vitamin C*

Table 12. The Amino Acids:
Our Natural Pharmacy (*Continued*)

Isoleucine and Leucine

Are involved in stress, energy, and muscle metabolism. Leucine stimulates insulin release and inhibits protein breakdown. Both are useful in stress states of surgery, trauma, cirrhosis, fever, and starvation.

Lysine

Controls viral infections; inhibits growth and recurrence of herpes complex; stimulates secretion of gastric juices; controls muscle contractions, spastic disorders.

Methionine

Removes excess brain histamine that can cause depression and compulsive/obsessiveness; prevents deposits and cohesion of fats in the liver; acts as memory builder by synthesizing choline.
Warnings:

- *Must be taken with vitamin B_6*
- *Avoid if you are manic-depressive or if you have low histamine levels*

Ornithine

May reduce fat and increase muscle mass by promoting fat metabolism and stimulating production of growth hormone; helps detoxify ammonia.

D-Phenylalanine

Controls pain; elevates moods by increasing endorphins.
Warning: Should not be taken by those with high blood pressure or anyone taking MAO inhibitors for depression.

L-Phenylalanine

Helps manage certain types of depression by increasing levels of the neurotransmitter norepinephrine, a precursor of epinephrine (adrenaline); increases blood pressure in individuals with low blood pressure.

Warnings:

- *Should not be used by anyone taking MAO inhibitors for depression*
- *Do not take if you have high blood pressure*

Proline

Can help lower blood pressure; promotes wound healing.

Serine

A derivative of glycine; can cause psychotic reactions and elevated blood pressure. No role has yet been developed for this amino acid.

Taurine

Can help inhibit epileptic seizures; helps repair muscle and tendon damage; helps promote skin flexibility, stops alcohol-withdrawal tremors.

Tryptophan

Helps alleviate depression by increasing levels of the neurotransmitter serotonin; induces sleep; has an antianxiety effect; appears to aid in blood clotting. Deficiency causes insomnia, depression.

Should be taken with vitamin B_6 and fruit juice to maximize uptake by the brain.

Tyrosine

Useful in combatting depression because it is a precursor of the neurotransmitters norepinephrine and adrenaline; is a precursor of thyroid hormone.

Warning: Should not be used by anyone taking a MAO inhibitor for depression or by those with malignant melanoma.

Table 12. The Amino Acids:
Our Natural Pharmacy (*Continued*)

Valine

Promotes muscle coordination and proper functioning of the nervous system; promotes mental vigor. Low serum valine is consistently found in patients with anorexia nervosa.

Amino Acids to
Serve Your Special Needs

You can already appreciate some of the remarkable properties of amino acids. By now you have firsthand experience with glutamine and its amazing ability to control cravings for alcohol and sugar. You are taking DL-phenylalanine to promote alertness, lift depression, elevate mood, and control pain by restoring brain levels of endorphins. And, of course, your adjusted nutrient plan contains a blend of eighteen amino acids in their purest form to provide you with all the essential precursors needed for neurotransmitter formation. These free-form amino acids have been treated so that your body can absorb and use them completely—even at this early stage of recovery when you may be short on the digestive acids and enzymes required for normal absorption. (Incidentally, the protein powders promoted as a means of building muscle mass do not provide predigested amino acids and cannot be substituted for the totally absorbable amino acids recommended here.)

Building on this base, we can add other amino acids and their cofactors—the nutrients needed to ensure that the amino acids are properly absorbed and utilized—to address your specific symptoms.

Figure 8, How Brain Chemicals Create Emotions, illustrates the relationship between brain chemicals, moods, and behavior. It isn't surprising that alcoholics whose neurotransmitters have been seriously altered by heavy alcohol use often complain of some of the following symptoms:

• Anxiety
• High stress, tension

Figure 8. How Brain Chemicals Create Emotions

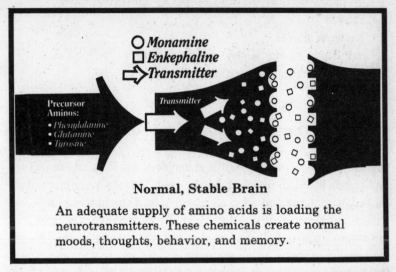

Normal, Stable Brain

An adequate supply of amino acids is loading the neurotransmitters. These chemicals create normal moods, thoughts, behavior, and memory.

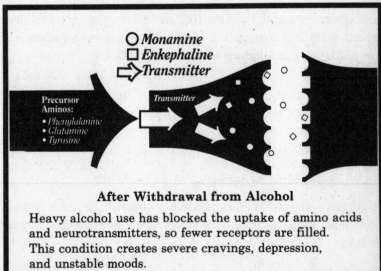

After Withdrawal from Alcohol

Heavy alcohol use has blocked the uptake of amino acids and neurotransmitters, so fewer receptors are filled. This condition creates severe cravings, depression, and unstable moods.

- Short-term memory loss
- Insomnia
- Fatigue
- Tremors, shakes
- Irritability, sudden anger, violent outbursts
- Poor concentration, high distractability
- Depression

The HRC Replacement Formulas

On the following pages you'll find replacement formulas for all the complaints listed above. Each will be preceded by a description of the formula's contents and an explanation of how the nutrients will contribute to your recovery. All the ingredients are perfectly safe. They are amino acids and other natural chemicals essential to your health. No formula contains drugs of any type. I can testify with great confidence to their safety and effectiveness. All of the formulas have been carefully tested and used in the HRC treatment program for the past several years. For information about obtaining these formulas, call BIO-RECOVERY in Minneapolis at 1-800-24-SOBER.

Anxiety

The HRC formula for anxiety (Table 13) includes the calming amino acids GABA and tryptophan plus vitamins and minerals noted for their soothing effects:

GABA (Gamma-Aminobutyric Acid):

GABA has a powerful calming effect on the brain. In fact, tranquilizers like Valium and Librium work by stimulating the brain's receptors for GABA.

Tryptophan:

This precursor of the sleep-inducing neurotransmitter serotonin also has relaxing and calming effects. Serotonin levels are often low among people with anxiety disorders. A recent study found that 44 percent of alcoholics suffer from anxiety. You can be pretty sure that you are

Table 13. The HRC Formula for Anxiety

Nutrient	Dose	Directions
GABA**	100 mg	2 capsules 4 times per day
L-Tryptophan*†**	500 mg	1 capsule 3 times per day
Histidine**	500 mg	1 capsule 2 times per day
Chromium picolinate*	200 mcg	1 capsule per day
Niacinamide	500 mg	1 capsule 3 times per day
Vitamin C*	1,000 mg	1 capsule 3 times per day
Vitamin B$_6$*	200 mg	1 capsule 3 times per day
Vitamin E*	200 IU	1 capsule 3 times per day

*This level was partly or completely established in your adjusted nutrient plan or in other formulas you may be taking. Refer to your nutrient replacement list (Chart 6 or 7) to determine whether you need to add more of this nutrient to achieve the level suggested here.
†Use tryptophan only if the FDA lifts the current ban on its sale.
**Warnings: Do not take histidine if lab tests show that your blood histamine levels are elevated.
  Your total daily dose of GABA, tryptophan, and histidine should not exceed the amounts contained in this formula.

low on tryptophan if you have ever blacked out from drinking. It has been established that low tryptophan stores trigger blackouts.

You will also be taking chromium picolinate to promote conversion of tryptophan to serotonin. It accomplishes this by facilitating absorption into muscle tissue of the amino acids that compete with tryptophan for access to the brain.

Histidine:

This amino acid is converted in the brain to histamine, which reduces the intensity of the brain waves underlying anxiety, confusion, and irritability and raises the level of the brain waves that relax and calm by strengthening alpha-wave activity.

WARNING: *Do not take histidine if lab tests show that your blood histamine levels are elevated.*

Other Nutrients:

In addition to the amino acids discussed above, certain B vitamins are crucial to reducing anxiety. Indeed, the textbook description of anxiety neurosis exactly matches the symptoms of vitamin B_3 (niacin) deficiency: hyperactivity, depression, fatigue, apprehension, headache, and insomnia. A deficiency of vitamin B_6 (pyridoxine) causes extreme anxiety, nervousness, confusion, and melancholy. Vitamin B_6 is easily destroyed by heavy use of alcohol, drugs, and refined sugars.

Can B vitamins relieve anxiety? An interesting new study showed significantly decreased levels of anxiety among a group of alcoholics treated with megavitamins. Over a twenty-one-day period, the group took approximately three grams of vitamin C, three grams of niacin, six hundred milligrams of B_6 and six hundred international units (IU) of vitamin E per day. A comparison group received only inert gelatin capsules. None of the subjects in either group took antidepressants or antianxiety drugs. Anxiety levels among both groups were measured three times over the twenty-one days. They fell dramatically *only* in the group on megavitamin therapy.

In people with chronic anxiety unrelated to life events, an injection of sodium lactate will trigger a panic attack. Eating a lot of foods high in refined sugar increases blood lactate levels and can induce panic in susceptible persons. The chromium picolinate in the HRC anxiety formula stabilizes blood sugar and helps prevent panic. Eliminating caffeine and alcohol and refined sugars from the diet is essential for anyone suffering from anxiety.

Stress

I have already discussed the amazing power of pantothenic acid to reduce stress. Remember those prison volunteers who became irritable, tense, sullen, quarrelsome, and depressed when fed a diet deficient in pantothenic acid? You won't be surprised to learn that the HRC formula for stress (Table 14) includes pantothenic acid, B_5, which combats stress by rebuilding adrenal glands exhausted by alcoholism.

Other stress fighters include glutamine, which rids the body of ammonia that builds up as a result of the protein destruction brought on by stress. Two now-familiar amino acids, phenylalanine and tyro-

Table 14. The HRC Formula for Stress

Nutrient	Dose	Directions
Glutamine*	500 mg	2 capsules 3 times per day
Phenylalanine*	500 mg	1 capsule 2 times per day
Tyrosine*	500 mg	1 capsule 2 times per day
Pantothenic acid†	500 mg	2 capsules per day
Vitamin C*	1,000 mg	1 capsule 3 times per day
B Complex†	50 mg	1 capsule 3 times per day
Zinc*	20 mg	1 capsule 2 times a day

*The level of pantothenic acid was partly established in your adjusted nutrient plan.
†You are already taking this amount as part of your adjusted nutrient plan. Do not duplicate.
**Your multivitamin/mineral capsules already provide sufficient B-complex vitamins. Do not duplicate dose. However, they do *not* supply enough pantothenic acid.

sine, help in other ways. Phenylalanine is converted into adrenaline to replenish supplies exhausted by stress. Tyrosine combined with iodine from the salt in your diet will help your thyroid form the hormone thyroxine, which lessens stress by stabilizing your metabolic rate.

Vitamin C is also a potent stress fighter that works with pantothenic acid to rebuild the adrenal glands. You also will be taking B-complex vitamins to soothe your nerves and boost your energy. The formula also includes zinc to help you absorb the B vitamins.

With the exception of pantothenic acid and tyrosine, all of the levels of nutrients specified in the HRC stress formula are already part of your daily nutrient program. I am providing you with the stress formula for future use. There may come a time when stress threatens your sobriety. Should that happen, begin taking the formula as directed and continue for one month.

Memory Loss

Is your short-term memory failing? Alcohol is probably responsible. Gary Tollefson, Ph.D., a medical researcher at the University of Minnesota, came up with some striking findings about memory loss among alcoholics. He compared the postmortem brains of people who suffered from memory loss in old age with those of heavy drinkers. He found that the brain cells of alcoholics—specifically, the structures involving memory processing—age prematurely. The most seriously affected are tissues within the hippocampus, a segment of the brain responsible for the initial processing of long-term memory and storage of short-term recall.

Tollefson's study focused on acetylcholine, a neurotransmitter that plays a key role in short-term memory. Alcoholics as well as the elderly suffer gradual loss of this vital neurotransmitter. The brain compensates for this change by heightening the sensitivity of the receptors carrying memory messages, but because of the acetylcholine shortage, the transmission cannot be completed and short-term recall is poor.

Recovering alcoholics must resupply the precursor chemical—phosphatidylcholine, which is converted to acetylcholine in the brain and restores memory function. Other researchers have found that increasing dietary choline raises brain levels of acetylcholine. We use Twin Laboratories' PC55 phosphatidylcholine (from Germany), which has a 55 percent conversion rate, the highest available today. You will also be taking pantothenic acid, which is needed to convert phosphatidylcholine to acetylcholine (Table 15).

Two other nutrients—vitamin B_1 (thiamine) and vitamin B_{12} (cobalamine)—can help. Alcohol blocks absorption of thiamine, causing memory loss, central-nervous-system damage, and poor concentration. Obviously, you have to resupply this important nutrient. And you need B_{12} because concentration and memory difficulties can develop when this nutrient is unavailable or poorly absorbed.

Insomnia

A number of nutrients can calm you and help you sleep. Unfortunately, the best of all is tryptophan, which is unavailable in the United States at this time. In the brain, tryptophan is converted to the neurotransmitter serotonin, which causes us to fall sleep. Depletion of tryptophan as a result of heavy drinking explains why alcoholics suffer from insomnia.

Table 15. The HRC Formula for Memory Loss

Nutrient	Dose	Directions
Phosphatidylcholine (PC55, Twin Laboratories)	2 heaping tablespoons	take daily in juice or applesauce
Pantothenic acid*	500 mg	1 capsule per day
Vitamin B₁*	100 mg	3 capsules per day
Vitamin B₁₂*	500 mcg dots (Twin Laboratories)	dissolve 1 dot under the tongue at breakfast and another at dinner

*This level was partly or completely established in your adjusted nutrient plan or in other formulas you may be taking. Refer to your nutrient replacement list (Chart 6 or 7) to determine whether you need to add more of this nutrient to achieve the level suggested here.

Luckily, a number of other nutrients also have calming properties (Table 16). Inositol has a soothing effect on spinal-cord nerves, the brain, and cerebrospinal fluid and produces antianxiety effects similar to the drugs Librium and meprobamate. The amino-acid derivative GABA (gamma-aminobutyric acid) is also a calming substance. A formula called GABA Plus from Twin Laboratories combines inositol, GABA, and niacinamide to enhance sleep.

Vitamin B₆ (pyridoxine) is responsible for our dreams. Everyone dreams; if you have no dream recall, don't assume you have stopped dreaming. Begin taking additional vitamin B₆ every morning, and you will soon enjoy vivid technicolor dreams. The quality of your sleep will improve, too.

Vitamin C also promotes restful sleep. A study measuring possible brain and central-nervous-system stimulants and sedatives demonstrated that vitamin C has potent sedative, antianxiety properties.

The magnesium deficiencies so common among chronic alcoholics contribute to insomnia as well as restlessness, changes in heart rhythm, and tremors.

Table 16. The HRC Formula for Insomnia

Nutrient	Dose	Directions
L-Tryptophan*†	500 mg	2 to 5 capsules at bedtime with fruit juice
GABA Plus (Twin Laboratories):		1 to 4 capsules at bedtime
GABA*	100 mg	
Inositol*	600 mg	
Niacinamide*	300 mg	
Vitamin B$_6$* **	100 mg	1 capsule 3 times per day with meals
Vitamin C*	1,000 mg	1 capsule 3 times per day with meals

*This level was partly or completely established in your adjusted nutrient plan or in other formulas you may be taking. Refer to your nutrient replacement list (Chart 6 or 7) to determine whether you need to add more of this nutrient to achieve the level suggested here.
†Use tryptophan only if the FDA lifts the current ban on its sale.
**Warning: Increase the dose of B$_6$ until dream recall occurs. Do not exceed 700 mg per day unless you are pyroluric (kryptopyrolles block uptake of B$_6$, in which case you will need 1,000 mg or more daily).

Calcium is essential for controlling the excitability of the nervous system. It has a calming effect that will help you sleep normally.

Fatigue

Much of the chronic fatigue and exhaustion experienced by alcoholics may stem from overstressed and exhausted adrenal glands. Endocrinologist John Tintera, M.D., whose work I have described in earlier chapters, notes that the most common symptom of hypoadrenocorticism (failing adrenals) is monumental fatigue and loss of stamina. This state of exhaustion can be reversed only by carefully adhering to a diet to counteract hypoglycemia and rebuilding the adrenal glands.

Dr. Tintera treated this condition with a bovine adrenocortical extract injected intravenously over a period of several weeks. For a short time after the injection, the body of the recipient acknowledges the presence of this bovine adrenaline and lets its own adrenals rest and recuperate. I had personal experience with these injections during the early 1970s. At the time, a 17-keto steroid test showed that my adrenal glands were exhausted, probably from the stress of widowhood and single parenting. Fortunately, my physician knew about adrenocortical extract (ACE) and did not make the mistake of prescribing cortisone, which is a hundred times stronger. Cortisone is a synthetic drug powerful enough to completely take over adrenal function. If this happens, the adrenals can gradually atrophy. The longer you take cortisone, the lower your odds of getting off it and rebuilding your own adrenals. The drug also has some very undesirable side effects. It causes the face to round to a characteristic moon shape and alters the upper back into a "buffalo hump." Mental instability is another potential side effect. For these reasons, treatment with ACE is much safer. Another advantage is that ACE contains all the adrenocortical hormones, while cortisone contains only one—in a strength great enough to disrupt natural corticosteroid balance.

Today, few doctors inject ACE. However, you can get ACE drops. Placed under the tongue they are absorbed directly into the bloodstream. Our supplier is Ominopathy Products, 414 North State College Boulevard, Anaheim, CA 92806.

In addition to ACE, a number of nutrients will help you combat fatigue (Table 17). Glutamine can boost your energy by supplying adequate brain glucose, which prevents the mild insulin shock so common among hypoglycemic alcoholics. And Aminoplex, the free-form amino acid blend you take as part of your adjusted nutrient plan, can help restore the body's metabolic energy.

Pantothenic acid and vitamin C are also essential for restoration of adrenal health. Interestingly, native Americans used to eat animal adrenal glands in the winter, which gave them a supply of vitamin C until fruits and vegetables became available in the spring. Pantothenic acid is important for formation of the actual adrenocortical hormones.

You will also be taking B-complex vitamins to replenish deficiencies that can underlie fatigue. For example, a deficiency of B_1 (thiamine) causes fatigue; lack of B_2 (riboflavin) can make you sluggish; B_3 (niacin) deficiency causes your energy level to suffer; low B_{12} levels

Table 17. The HRC Formula for Fatigue

Nutrient	Dose	Directions
Glutamine*	500 mg	2 capsules mid-morning and 2 mid-afternoon
Free-form amino acids, Aminoplex, (Tyson)*	750 mg	2 capsules mid-morning and 2 mid-afternoon
Adrenocortical extract	2 sublingual drops	2 drops 3 times per day
Pantothenic acid*	500 mg	2 capsules per day
Vitamin C*	1,000 mg	1 capsule 3 times per day
B complex†	50 mg	1 capsule 3 times per day

*This level was partly or completely established in your adjusted nutrient plan or in other formulas you may be taking. Refer to your nutrient replacement list (Chart 6 or 7) to determine whether you need to add more of this nutrient to achieve the level suggested here.
†Your multivitamin/mineral capsules already provide sufficient B-complex vitamins. Do not duplicate dose.

can cause fatigue. And you need vitamin B_6 for proper adrenal functioning.

Pain Control

A number of studies have demonstrated that amino acids are extremely effective for relief of chronic pain. In one, oral doses of D-phenylalanine (not L-phenylalanine) provided significant relief for patients with lower back pain and chronic pain from lumbar fusion, neuralgia, and osteoarthritis. In another, two grams of D-phenylalanine taken one hour before a dental procedure resulted in a marked rise in the patient's pain threshold. Adding D-phenylalanine to morphine can reduce and, in some cases, eliminate individual variation in the drug's effectiveness. The explanation for these remarkable effects is the action of D-phenylalanine in the brain, where it appears to block the action of certain enzymes that normally break down and destroy endorphins and enkephalins, the body's natural painkillers. Three

Table 18. The HRC Formula for Pain

Nutrient	Dose	Directions
D-Phenylalanine	500 mg	2 capsules in the morning; 2 in the afternoon or evening on an empty stomach
L-Tryptophan*†	500 mg	2 capsules 3 times per day on an empty stomach
Vitamin B$_6$*	100 mg	1 or 2 capsules per day with food
Vitamin C*	1,000 mg	1 capsule 3 times per day with meals
Vitamin B$_3$ (non-time-released niacin)*	500 mg	1 capsule per day with food

*This level was partly or completely established in your adjusted nutrient plan or in other formulas you may be taking. Refer to your nutrient replacement list (Chart 6 or 7) to determine whether you need to add more of this nutrient to achieve the level suggested here.
†Use tryptophan only if the FDA lifts the current ban on its sale.

grams of D-phenylalanine has also proved effective for the control of bone-cancer pain.

Tryptophan can also help combat intractable pain as a result of its effect on the brain's primary pain-inhibiting center. For some people, three grams of tryptophan per day can reduce chronic maxillofacial pain. A study at the Massachusetts Institute of Technology found that three and a half grams of tryptophan decreased sensitivity to pain and increased drowsiness but did not impair sensorimotor performance. The cofactors vitamin C, niacin (vitamin B$_3$), and vitamin B$_6$ must be present for the tryptophan to be effective.

Alcohol-Induced Tremors, Shakiness

In a study of abstinent alcoholics, all of the participants continued to suffer from tremors ten weeks after treatment. This common problem can be reversed by combining the amino acid taurine with magnesium, calcium, B-complex vitamins, and omega-6 essential fatty acid (Table 19). Of these nutrients, the one that is new to you is taurine, which, according to a 1977 study, effectively blocked the shakes of alcohol withdrawal.

Omega-6 essential fatty acid (Efamol) can also reduce tremors that occur during alcohol withdrawal. This fatty acid is also essential to the prevention and treatment of alcohol-induced central-nervous-system impairment. Calcium and B-complex vitamins also help control this problem. All the B vitamins are essential to nervous-system stability, while calcium and magnesium calm and relax nerve tissue. The depletion of both these minerals by alcohol is responsible for the acute tremors that occur during withdrawal. It has been shown that magnesium can reverse delirium tremens. At Health Recovery Center we administer intravenous magnesium to control patients' muscle tremors and help prevent convulsive seizures.

Table 19. The HRC Formula for Tremors, Shakiness

Nutrient	Dose	Directions
Taurine	500 mg	1 capsule between breakfast and lunch; another between lunch and dinner
Calcium/magnesium*	300/150 mg	2 capsules 3 times per day with meals
B complex†	50 mg	1 capsule 3 times per day with meals
Efamol*	500 mg	2 capsules 3 times per day with meals

*This level was partly or completely established in your adjusted nutrient plan or in other formulas you may be taking. Refer to your nutrient replacement list (Chart 6 or 7) to determine whether you need to add more of this nutrient to achieve the level suggested here.
†Your multivitamin/mineral capsules already provide sufficient B-complex vitamins. Do not duplicate dose.

What About Emotions?

With few exceptions, we have concentrated in this chapter on physical symptoms. But some of the most painful problems recovering alcoholics face are the out-of-control emotions that can undermine their recovery. In the next chapter you will find formulas to help you with such difficulties as aggression, lack of concentration, and Wernicke-Korsakoff syndrome, a very serious psychiatric disorder that affects longtime alcoholics. You will also learn more about the nutrients you need to recover and maintain your health.

So far, I haven't mentioned depression. Because two-thirds of all alcoholics suffer from this potentially life-threatening disorder, you may be disappointed that I have not yet given you an antidepression formula. I won't disappoint you. This is a subject very close to my heart. As a result of my son's suicide, I have always paid special attention to the puzzle of alcoholic depression. The biochemical aspects of this mystery are far too complex for a simple formula. At HRC we have found that at least seven different biochemical patterns can underlie depression. All seven stem from alcohol-related changes in the biochemistry of the brain, not from responses to external events. It is essential to identify and address the physical damage that has given rise to these symptoms.

Chapter 10 is all about depression. It will help you identify the cause of your particular problem. Armed with the appropriate clues, you'll be able to undertake repair. But first let's move on to Chapter 9 and more formulas to speed your recovery.

Nine

Week Four:
Continuing Repair

By now your repair program should be paying big dividends. You are feeling better and have weaned your body away from alcohol—the addictive bond has been broken. Or has it? You may be physically free of your addiction to alcohol but still emotionally vulnerable to its grasp.

In Chapter 8 we discussed the physical basis for some of the emotional problems common among alcoholics. You won't be surprised to learn that a number of other emotional problems are caused by alcohol's depletion of the natural brain chemicals needed for stable emotions and good mental health. On the following pages I'll discuss aggression and irritability, short attention span or poor concentration, and Wernicke-Korsakoff syndrome, a serious psychiatric disorder seen in advanced alcoholism.

At the end of this chapter you will find tables that summarize your vitamin and mineral needs. Look them over carefully. Although this program provides you with adequate amounts of the vitamins and minerals alcohol depletes, after studying the tables you may feel that you need even more than you are getting. If so, you can increase the amount you take up to the therapeutic dose listed on the chart. But first scan your nutrient replacement list to double-check the amount you already take. Be sure not to exceed the therapeutic dose at any time. Enter any additional amounts on your tally sheet, but never, I repeat NEVER, exceed the therapeutic dose listed on the chart.

Now let's take a look at the emotional problems that can sabotage your recovery and discuss what you can do to overcome them.

HRC Replacement Formulas for Emotional Stability

Aggression, Irritability, Sudden Anger, Violent Outbursts

Years ago when I was new to this field, I represented our public-sector agency at a meeting with representatives of the local court system to discuss the many cases of verbal and physical abuse among alcoholics, drinking or sober. Several of the social workers present remarked that violence often continued whether or not the alcoholics had been treated or had stopped drinking on their own. The social workers felt that the outbursts were the result of personality traits common to many alcoholics. At the time, I wasn't familiar with the research linking brain chemistry and aggression, particularly the violence brought on by the hypoglycemic episodes experienced by so many alcoholics, regardless of whether or not they are drinking.

I later learned of some anthropological studies done in the 1970s among the Quolla Indians of Central America. Since the sixteenth century, the Quollas have been known for their violence; unpremeditated murder is rather common among them. The anthropologists discovered that Quolla diets were very poor: high in refined sugars and alcohol and short on basic nutrition. Every single one of the tribesmen tested turned out to be hypoglycemic. What's more, the most violent of the Indians had supernormal surges of adrenaline when their glucose levels fell too low.

By now you know enough about hypoglycemia to understand what can happen under these circumstances. By the time the adrenaline is released, the reasoning brain has turned off, leaving the animal brain in charge. At best, this abnormal situation can erupt in verbal anger. At worst, it can bring on physical aggression that can have tragic results. Consider this depressingly familiar scenario: an abusive spouse leaves a favorite bar in a hypoglycemic state brought on by an evening of heavy drinking and arrives home about the time the adrenaline hits the bloodstream. At this point, anyone unfortunate enough to cross his or her path may be subjected to uncontrollable anger expressed as physical abuse. Counseling has little to offer these people. Our prisons are full of such violent hypoglycemics.

If hypoglycemic alcoholics stop drinking but continue to consume large amounts of caffeine and refined sugars, the outbursts of irritability and sudden anger will continue. These symptoms will disappear only when brain glucose levels stabilize. For me, one of the most gratifying results of the HRC repair program is the immense relief clients report when their anger disappears.

Some other enlightening findings on the chemistry of violence and anger come from a 1982 study of two groups of murderers. The first group had committed unprovoked murders; their aggression was deemed spontaneous. The second group was labeled paranoid and had killed only after much premeditation. An analysis of the cerebrospinal fluid of both groups revealed that levels of a serotonin metabolite (hydroxyindoleactic acid or 5HIAA) were significantly lower among the unprovoked, spontaneous murderers than either the paranoid group or a group of normal noncriminal controls.

Since serotonin is derived from tryptophan, we can conclude that calm, nonviolent brain chemistry requires an adequate intake of tryptophan plus vitamins B_3 and B_6, the nutrients needed to promote conversion of tryptophan to serotonin.

Another brain chemical with calming properties is gamma-aminobutyric acid, better known as GABA. You may be interested to know that tranquilizers like Valium and Ativan owe their soothing effects to the fact that they stimulate GABA receptors in the brain. You can get the same effect with a formula called Calm Kids, manufactured by Natrol. At HRC we have found that this formula also works well for adults (Table 20). Six capsules per day provide eight hundred milligrams of GABA. This calming formula also contains

- Glycine, an amino acid that can reduce aggression when combined with the vitamin inositol
- Taurine, another amino acid, which helps regulate the excitable tissues of the central nervous system
- Herbal passion flower extract, a formulation that also has a calming influence on the brain
- Vitamin C
- Calcium
- Vitamin B$_6$ (Pyridoxine)
- Magnesium

Table 20. The HRC Formula for Aggression, Irritability, Sudden Anger

Nutrient	Dose/Capsule	Directions
L-Tryptophan*†	500 mg	1 capsule 3 times per day between meals
Vitamin B$_6$ (pyridoxal-5^1-phosphate)*	3.3 mg	1 capsule per day
Niacin*	500 mg	1 capsule per day
Calm Kids (Natrol)**		2 capsules 3 times per day
GABA	133 mg	
Glycine	133 mg	
Taurine	83 mg	
Passion flower	83 mg	
Vitamin C	10 mg	
Calcium	16.6 mg	
Magnesium	8.3 mg	
Vitamin B$_6$ (pyridoxine)	8.3 mg	

*This level was partly or completely established in your adjusted nutrient plan or in other formulas you may be taking. Refer to your nutrient replacement list (Chart 6 or 7) to determine whether you need to add more of this nutrient to achieve the level suggested here.
†Use tryptophan only if the FDA lifts the current ban on its sale.
**Do not add the nutrients in Calm Kids to your nutrient replacement list.

You do not have to add the nutrients in Calm Kids to the totals on your nutrient replacement list.

Poor Concentration, Short Attention Span

Many alcoholics trace their difficulties with concentration back to childhood. These people also tend to be fidgety, easily distracted, impulsive, and clumsy. Some say they became addicted to marijuana because it calms them. If this is your problem, you may have an undiscovered food allergy. There is also the possibility that the toxic effects on the brain of the many additives, chemicals, and dyes in our foods may be to blame.

A number of studies have linked hyperactivity and other childhood problems to food additives. There is also some persuasive circumstantial evidence to support this connection. In Europe, where less than twenty food additives are approved for use, hyperactivity among children is comparatively rare, affecting only one child in two thousand, as compared to one in four in the United States, where more than four thousand food additives are in use.

Studies in Germany have shown that many children are highly sensitive to the phosphate (the bubbles) in soda pop. Researchers have found that phosphates can induce aggression and violence and may underlie handwriting changes and even dyslexia.

Doctors once believed that children outgrow hyperactivity in adolescence, but we now know that there is no magic age at which symptoms disappear. Many adults exhibit telltale signs of hyperactivity, including nervous habits such as nail biting and foot jiggling, workaholic habits, unstable emotions, insomnia, restless sleep, irritability, speaking with a louder or more highly pitched voice when stressed, and adult temper tantrums.

Without help, troubled children grow into equally troubled adults. They are sometimes disliked because of their aggressive, defiant personalities.

The root of these problems is often the effect of certain foods and chemicals on the formation of GABA, a calming neurotransmitter in the brain. An enzyme known as GAD (glutamic acid decarboxylase) is essential to normal GABA formation. We now know that GAD can be blocked or inhibited by a number of substances or conditions, including

- Food additives (artificial dyes)
- Salicylates, natural chemicals abundant in almonds, apples, apricots, berries, cherries, grapes, nectarines, oranges, peaches, plums, prunes, and raisins
- A low-protein diet
- Estrogens
- Oxidation
- Vitamin B_6 deficiency

Many of our clients have overcome hyperactivity, irritability, and poor concentration by taking GABA supplements. (We recommend that they also avoid chlorinated water, refined sugars, dyes, food additives, salicylates, and all foods and drugs containing caffeine or nicotine.)

The amino acid histidine aids in this repair process by reducing the intensity of the brain's beta waves (which promote alertness, cognitive thinking, and excitability) and by enhancing calming alpha waves.

Our HRC formula for high distractibility, short attention span, and poor concentration (Table 21) also contains some now-familiar ingredients.

Tryptophan helps boost the availability of the calming neurotransmitter serotonin.

The antioxidant complex helps protect you from the effects of environmental pollution (automobile exhaust, formaldehydes, cigarette smoke) as well as food dyes, additives, and chemicals that can trigger reactions in susceptible individuals.

Omega-6 essential fatty acid (Efamol) has also proven useful. Some compelling scientific evidence links a lack of essential fatty acids to hyperactivity. An English study of ten thousand hyperactive youngsters detected consistent abnormalities in essential fatty acid availability. The findings were challenged by two groups of New Zealand psychiatrists; they tested hyperactive children themselves and came up with the same results: inadequate availability of omega-6 essential fatty acids.

Table 21. The HRC Formula for High Distractibility, Short Attention Span, Poor Concentration

Nutrient	Dose	Directions
Histidine*	500 mg	1 capsule per day ½ hour before a meal
L-Tryptophan*†	500 mg	1 capsule 3 times per day, ½ hour before each meal
Antioxidant complex*		1 capsule per day
Efamol*	500 mg	2 capsules 3 times per day with meals
Calm Kids (Natrol)**		6 capsules per day

*This level was partly or completely established in your adjusted nutrient plan or in other formulas you may be taking. Refer to your nutrient replacement list (Chart 6 or 7) to determine whether you need to add more of this nutrient to achieve the level suggested here.
†Use tryptophan only if the FDA lifts the current ban on its sale.
**See Table 20 for a description of this formula. Do not add the nutrients in Calm Kids to your nutrient replacement list.

Further evidence comes from Paul Wender, M.D., a Salt Lake City epidemiologist who correlated childhood hyperactivity with a higher than normal risk of alcoholism later in life. The underlying chemistry here is a bit tricky to follow: a lack of essential fatty acids is one of several factors that cause defects in a component of the immune system, the T suppressor lymphocytes. When these T suppressors fail to function properly, allergic reactions develop. Among these reactions is the classic allergic/addicted response to the grains in alcohol. Replacing omega-6 essential fatty acid will help improve T suppressor cell functioning, which in turn enhances control over allergic reactions.

Wernicke-Korsakoff Syndrome

Wernicke-Korsakoff syndrome stems from causes similar to those of beriberi, depletion of the body's stores of thiamine (vitamin B_1) from many years of malnutrition due to alcoholism. Symptoms include anemia, anxiety, depression, and confusion. About 40 percent of those affected also have anemia as a result of folic acid deficiency. At HRC, we treat Wernicke-Korsakoff syndrome with weekly injections of thiamine. Clients also take daily doses of thiamine in capsule form (Table 22).

Korsakoff's psychosis, a disorder stemming from destruction of nerve fibers connecting brain cells, is a serious neurological/psychiatric disorder seen in advanced alcoholism. It stems from the effects of the acetaldehyde that builds up in the liver and spills over into the bloodstream, where it creates free radicals that cause damage throughout the body. In the brain it can impair cellular communication by injuring the nerve fibers connecting cells. The prescription drug Hydergine stimulates regrowth of these damaged nerve fibers. The most effective form of Hydergine comes in tablets, which can be placed under the tongue for immediate absorption. Ask your doctor about Hydergine if you feel you need help in this area.

Table 22. The HRC Formula for Wernicke-Korsakoff Syndrome

Nutrient	Dose	Directions
Thiamine (vitamin B$_1$)*†	600 mg	2 capsules 3 times per day with meals
Hydergine**	up to 10 mg daily	Place sublingual tablets under tongue as prescribed

*This level was partly or completely established in your adjusted nutrient plan or in other formulas you may be taking. Refer to your nutrient replacement list (Chart 6 or 7) to determine whether you need to add more of this nutrient to achieve the level suggested here.
†An injection of 100 mg of thiamine once or twice a week will speed repair. Consult your physician.
**Must be prescribed by your physician.

Supernutrition:
Personalizing Your Recovery Strategy

Now it's time to get really personal. You already know that alcohol depletes your body of many essential nutrients, causing both physical and mental changes. Your repair program is restoring key nutrients and, by now, you almost certainly have noticed a major improvement in the way you feel. At this point, you are going to fine-tune your program by assessing your nutritional status. If you have any physical or emotional symptoms that could be related to a vitamin or mineral deficiency, you can adjust your nutrient intake to correct matters.

I already have mentioned that lab tests are not always the best way to diagnose nutritional deficiencies. These tests tell you about levels of nutrients circulating in your blood but don't reveal what's going on at the cellular level. The way you feel can be a better measure of your nutritional status than any blood test.

Alcohol depletes many nutrients, causing serious deficiencies; apart from that general statement, all I can tell you is that individual biochemical and genetic factors determine how quickly or slowly deficiencies develop. Some can occur even in the very early stages of alcoholism. Vitamin requirements vary enormously. The minimum daily allowances may be adequate for people in good health; megadoses are often needed by alcoholics suffering from acute malnutrition.

Vitamins and minerals are natural substances and are not toxic like drugs. Of course, at very high levels *any* substance—even water—can be harmful to your body. That is why you are keeping track of the amounts you are taking. They are found in the foods we eat, and we rely upon them to support life. Our bodies cannot for the most part manufacture these essential nutrients. Serious vitamin, mineral, and amino acid deficiencies can bring on major physical and emotional problems.

Some dieticians erroneously believe that alcoholics can immediately restore depleted levels of nutrients by "eating right." I wish it were that simple. Since alcohol disturbs the *process* by which our bodies absorb nutrients, alcoholics have to oversupply their systems until normal absorption resumes. Unfortunately, just "eating right" won't give you enough nutrients. Years of drinking can so disrupt normal intestinal processes that your liver can no longer properly absorb nutrients from the bloodstream. To make matters worse, alcohol-induced liver damage can limit this organ's capacity to store essential nutrients.

These disruptions can wreak havoc with an alcoholic's nutritional status. In one study, all the alcoholics participating were deficient in pantothenic acid. When Tao and Fox administered the vitamin orally, they found that the alcoholics couldn't absorb it—it was all excreted in the urine. With biochemical repair, these processes will revert to normal. However, it takes time. In the case of the alcoholics described above, it took ten weeks before they were able to absorb pantothenic acid properly.

Recently, I witnessed firsthand an example of how long it takes an alcoholic to recover from nutritional deficiencies. Harry's depression lifted when he took the amino acid tyrosine to restore the antidepressant neurotransmitter norepinephrine. He finished taking his first batch of tyrosine four weeks into the program and didn't replenish his supply. Within days, his depression returned. Harry needed more tyrosine to keep the depression at bay.

Keeping Track

You are now at the halfway mark of your repair program. Still to come are all-important formulas to help you banish depression, plus a discussion of how chemical sensitivities, food allergies, and *Candida albicans* overgrowth may be affecting your health. But now's a good time to check your progress. Read through the list below to make sure you are on schedule and that your repair program is progressing according to plan.

_____ You are following the Health Recovery Center diet for alcoholics.

_____ You are taking your adjusted nutrient plan formula.

_____ You have begun to exercise regularly. (The minimum requirement here is a brisk forty-five minute walk at least four times a week.)

Table 23. Vitamins

Vitamin	Symptoms of Deficiency	Symptoms of Toxicity	Found in	Recommended Daily Allowance (Adults)	Maximum Therapeutic Repair Dosage for Alcoholic Adults
A (Palmitate; Beta-Carotene)	Frequent colds, respiratory illness, calcium phosphate kidney stones, acne, dry skin, night blindness, burning eyes, eye infections, poor nails and dull hair, insomnia and fatigue	Aches and pains, poor appetite, yellowing of skin, weight loss, sore eyes, enlarged liver, decalcification of bones	Green leafy vegetables, liver, eggs, whole milk, cream, carrots, fruits, cod liver oil	6,000 IU adults 3,000 IU children	25,000 IU
B₁ (Thiamine)	Mental confusion, depression, fatigue, apathy, anxiety, inability to concentrate or tolerate pain,	Water soluble; excess is not stored in body	Dairy products, brewer's yeast, bran, mushrooms, dark green vegetables, organ meats	1 mg to 1.5 mg (0.5 mg per 1,000 calories of food)	300 mg daily

	sensitivity to noise, low blood pressure, heart palpitations, numbness or burning in hands and feet			
B_2 (Riboflavin)	Red tongue, cracks in corners of mouth, dizziness, watery or bloodshot eyes, hair loss, brain and nervous system changes, mental sluggishness, depression	Water soluble; excess is not stored in body	Dairy products, organ meats, brewer's yeast, poultry, fish, eggs, dried beans, peanuts	10 mg 100 mg

Table 23. Vitamins (Continued)

Vitamin	Symptoms of Deficiency	Symptoms of Toxicity	Found in	Recommended Daily Allowance (Adults)	Maximum Therapeutic Repair Dosage for Alcoholic Adults
B$_3$ (Niacin)	Fear, suspicion, depression, insomnia, weakness, irritability, mental confusion, red-tipped tongue, sore mouth, dermatitis, excessive gas	Large doses of niacin should be avoided by those with liver disease; may cause a marked drop in blood pressure; raises blood-sugar levels; can irritate ulcers because of its acidity; raises uric-acid levels and so can trigger gout	Lean meats, peanuts, brewer's yeast, wheat germ, desiccated liver, fish, poultry	18 mg (men) 13 mg (women)	100 mg to 3,000 mg
B$_5$ (Pantothenic Acid)	Fatigue, sleep disturbances, depression, adrenal exhaustion,	Water soluble; excess is not stored in the body	Organ meats, bran, peanuts, brewer's yeast	10 mg	100 mg to 1,000 mg

recurrent
respiratory
illness,
constipation, low
blood pressure,
irritability,
burning feet

	Deficiency Symptoms	Cautions	Food Sources	RDA	Therapeutic Dose
B$_6$ (Pyridoxine)	Mental confusion, irritability, depression, anxiety, numbness or cramping in hands and feet, insomnia, nausea in the morning, anemia, water retention, PMS symptoms	Extended use at levels over 1,000 mg has resulted in numbness of extremities	Meats, fish, peanuts, soybeans, bananas, whole grains, spinach, broccoli, legumes	2.2 mg	100 mg to 500 mg

Table 23. Vitamins (*Continued*)

Vitamin	Symptoms of Deficiency	Symptoms of Toxicity	Found in	Recommended Daily Allowance (Adults)	Maximum Therapeutic Repair Dosage for Alcoholic Adults
B_{12} (Cobalamin)	Pernicious anemia, neurological changes, numbness, poor reflexes, apathy, poor concentration, confusion, paranoia, poor memory	Water soluble; excess is not stored in the body	Eggs, meat, poultry, fish, dairy products, brewer's yeast	6 mcg	1,000 mcg (1 mg)
Folic Acid	Anemia, poor digestion, constipation, diarrhea, deterioration of nervous system, apathy, withdrawal,	Masks B_{12} pernicious anemia. Water soluble; excess is not stored in the body	Green leafy vegetables, wheat germ, dried beans and peas	400 mcg	800 mcg to 3 mg

	irritability, poor memory				
Choline	Low levels of phosphatidylcholine prevent adequate conversion to memory neurotransmitter (acetylcholine)	Unknown	Lecithin, egg yolks	None established	10 g daily to treat memory loss
Inositol	Poor sleep	Unknown	Whole grains, lecithin, liver, brewer's yeast	None established	100 mg to 1,000 mg (to sleep)
Biotin	Fatigue, depression, skin disorders, muscle pain	Unknown	Yeast, pork and lamb liver, egg yolk, nuts (especially peanuts)	None established (our own bodies make about 300 mg daily)	

Table 23. Vitamins (*Continued*)

Vitamin	Symptoms of Deficiency	Symptoms of Toxicity	Found in	Recommended Daily Allowance (Adults)	Maximum Therapeutic Repair Dosage for Alcoholic Adults
C	Fatigue, loss of appetite, sore gums, slow wound healing, aching joints, bruising easily, frequent infections, mental disorders	Rare; water soluble; high doses will eventually cause diarrhea; ascorbic acid form of vitamin C can activate peptic ulcer in susceptible people	Citrus fruits, cauliflower, brussels sprouts, broccoli	20 mg	3,000 mg to 6,000 mg daily; for alcohol withdrawal and detoxing, up to 25 g daily
D	Rickets, rheumatic pains, exhaustion, hypothyroidism	Calcium storage and calcification in the soft tissues of the body, frequent thirst and urination, nausea, vomiting, weakness, loss of appetite	Cod liver oil, sunlight, egg yolk, fish; frequently added to dairy products	400 IU	400 IU (consider the possibility of overdose because of the addition of vitamin D to many dairy products)

E	Restlessness, fatigue, insomnia, menopause symptoms, muscle wasting, liver damage	High blood pressure may occur if high doses are taken at outset of use	Wheat germ, cold-pressed oils (sunflower, safflower), spinach, broccoli, sweet potatoes, almonds, walnuts	15 IU	400 IU to 800 IU
K	Bleeding disorders, hemorrhaging	Natural K is not toxic	Leafy green vegetables, tomatoes, pork liver, carrots	None	500 mcg; antibiotics and sulfa drugs destroy K-containing intestinal bacteria; acidophilus culture 3 times daily replaces this friendly flora

Table 24. Minerals and Trace Elements

Mineral	Symptoms of Deficiency	Symptoms of Toxicity	Found in	Recommended Daily Allowance RDA (Adults)	Maximum Therapeutic Repair Dosage for Alcoholics
Calcium (Ca)	Leg and feet cramps, numbness, irritability, tenseness, insomnia, anxiety, nervousness, periodontal disease, osteoporosis	Bone and tissue calcification	Dairy products, almonds, sunflower seeds, parsley, bone meal, watercress, whole grains	800 mg	1,500 mg
Chromium (Cr)	Diabetes, hypoglycemia, heart disease	No oral toxicity ever reported	Brewer's yeast, meats, beef liver, shellfish, whole wheat, rye, butter, oysters, margarine, cornmeal, shrimp	10 mcg to 30 mcg	480 mcg
Copper (Cu)	Anemia, weakness, hypothyroidism	Paranoia, fears, hallucinations, aggressiveness, hyperactivity,	Oysters, Brazil nuts, soy lecithin, almonds, walnuts, beef liver, clams,	2 mg	1 mg to 3 mg

		stuttering, premature aging	cod liver oil, lamb, rye, butter, garlic		
Iron (Fe)	Anemia, dizziness, weakness, inability to concentrate, poor memory, depression	Bronzing of skin, liver toxicity, cardiac insufficiency	Kelp, brewers yeast, meats, eggs, green vegetables	10 mg (men) 20 mg (menstruating women)	Ferric citrate: up to 50 mg. (Supplement iron with E because E is destroyed by iron supplements)
Magnesium (Mg)	Memory impairment, insomnia, weakness, tremor, numbness, personality change, rapid heartbeat, hyperactivity, muscle aches, fatigue, anxiety, depression, delirium tremens	Drowsiness, stupor	Kelp, green leafy vegetables, peas, molasses, whole grains, soybeans, brown rice, almonds, cashews	350 mg	1,000 mg

Table 24. Minerals and Trace Elements (Continued)

Mineral	Symptoms of Deficiency	Symptoms of Toxicity	Found in	Recommended Daily Allowance RDA (Adults)	Maximum Therapeutic Repair Dosage for Alcoholics
Manganese (Mn)	Reduced levels of dopamine, slow bone healing, disc problems in the back, sore knees due to cartilage damage, impaired glucose tolerance, reduced brain function and inner-ear balance; severe deficiency produces skipped heartbeats and convulsions	Schizophrenic-like symptoms, tremor, muscular rigidity	Turnip greens, rhubarb, brussels sprouts, oatmeal, millet, cornmeal, carrots, eggs, pork and lamb, tomatoes, cantaloupe, whole-grain cereals	5 mg	20 mg
Potassium (K)	Muscle cramps, fatigue, weakness, constipation, edema, headache, heart arrhythmia, joint pain	Cardiac arrest, apathy; kidney failure or dehydration can elevate potassium to toxic levels	Oranges, dark green leafy vegetables, legumes, avocado, bananas, squash, tomatoes, sunflower seeds	2 g to 6 g	Usually not needed; can use lite salt or no salt to boost potassium intake

Mineral					
Selenium (Se)	Contributes to cancer and heart disease	Loss of hair and nails, paralysis, lassitude	Butter, smoked herring, wheat germ, bran, liver, eggs	50 to 200 mcg	300 mcg
Sodium (Na)	Low blood pressure, hot-weather weakness, weariness	Swelling, tension, irritability, high blood pressure, PMS symptoms	Kelp, green olives, dill pickles, cheddar cheese, table salt, soy sauce, potato chips	4 g	Not needed except for sunstroke or exhausted adrenals
Zinc (Zn)	Cold extremities, poor peripheral circulation, loss of taste, smell, poor wound healing, lethargy, poor appetite, prostate problems, acne, toxic copper levels, hypothyroidism	Drowsiness, vomiting, copper deficiency	Oysters, gingerroot, round steak, lamb, pecans, peas, shrimp, parsley, potatoes	15 mg	25 mg to 50 mg

_____ You are seeing your physician about any abnormal lab test results.

_____ You are cutting down on cigarettes. (In the next chapter, you'll get help with quitting.)

_____ You have found a support group (AA, Women for Sobriety) and/or have found friends who are recovering from this disease and understand and support you at this time.

Your persistence in following your recovery program will reap new rewards with every week. Congratulations for taking charge of your life with these positive steps.

Ten

Week Five:
Good-bye Depression

If you have been unsuccessfully battling depression, you are not alone. At least 40 percent of all alcoholics in the United States are affected. I say at least because our Health Recovery Center study found that almost two-thirds of our clients are depressed at entry. In fact, most alcoholics I have treated suffered from some degree of depression.

It is tempting to pin the blame for hopelessness and despair on the external events that can be triggered by alcoholism, such as the deterioration of a marriage or the loss of a job. To be sure, some of the depression alcoholics report is a result of the negative course life can take when you drink too much. You will be relieved to learn that this type of situational depression is self-limiting and will pass when your life begins to improve. Counseling or group therapy can be of enormous value here.

But depression among alcoholics usually runs much deeper than the situational variety I have just described. Depression, like the other emotional problems discussed in Chapter 8, often has biochemical roots that stem from the destructive effect of alcohol on the normal chemistry of the brain. Research has verified the relationship between biochemistry and depression. Autopsies of people who have committed suicide have revealed biochemical disruptions that may be unique to suicidal depression. In this chapter you will learn to recognize the warning signs of this tragedy in the making.

No amount of counseling or psychotherapy can help people who suffer from biochemically induced depression. I learned this the hard way, watching my son fight the deep sadness and feelings of hopelessness that descended upon him as his depression worsened. The counseling he received was excellent, but words have no power to reverse the biochemical disruption caused by alcoholism and drugs. In fact, therapy's focus on the unhappy or unsatisfactory external events marring the lives of such seriously depressed people only creates more misery.

My search for an explanation for Rob's suicide led me to studies that confirmed the connections between brain biochemistry and depression and offered methods of repair that work far more reliably than any form of talk therapy. I learned that there is no single biochemical glitch that explains all depression. At HRC, we treat seven different sources of depression that affect alcoholics. In this chapter, you will learn which of the seven may underlie your depression (in some cases, two or more may be to blame). You will also learn how to overcome your particular chemical problem or problems. This may mean taking even more nutrients. It may require further changes in your diet. Or you may need drug treatment to correct a medical condition that can precipitate depression. First, of course, you'll have to confirm that you are depressed. Then you can evaluate the severity of your case.

How Can You Tell if You Are Depressed?

Although two-thirds of the clients at HRC are severely depressed when they enter the program, many do not realize they are affected.

Men in particular are inclined to attribute the feelings induced by depression to other causes. Some blame their inability to handle stress well. Others reject being labeled depressed because of the social stigma often unjustly attached to this condition. Some are simply so overwhelmed by alcoholic symptoms that their depression is masked. Even so, depression is not difficult to spot if you know that certain behaviors are red flags to the condition:

- Withdrawal from activity; isolating yourself
- Continual fatigue, lethargy
- Indecisiveness
- Lack of motivation, boredom, loss of interest in life
- Feeling helpless, immobilized
- Sleeping too much; using sleep to escape reality
- Insomnia, particularly early morning insomnia (waking very early and being unable to get back to sleep)
- Lack of response to good news
- Loss of appetite or binge eating
- Ongoing anxiety
- Silent and unresponsive around people
- An "I don't care" attitude
- Easily upset or angered, lashing out at others
- Inability to concentrate
- Listening to mood music persistently
- Self-destructive behavior (including promiscuity)
- Suicidal thoughts or plans

How to Tell if Your Depression Is Psychological or Biochemical

Biochemical depression has certain symptoms that distinguish it from the depression stemming from negative life events. You have reason to suspect that you are biochemically depressed if any of the markers listed below describes your depression:

- You have been depressed for a long time despite changes in your life

- Talk therapy has little or no effect; in fact, psychological probing—questions like "Why do you hate your father?"—leave you as confused as Alice at the Mad Hatter's tea party
- You don't react to good news
- You awaken very early in the morning and can't get back to sleep
- You cannot trace the onset of your depression to any event in your life
- Your moods may swing between depression and elation over a period of months in a regular rhythm (this suggests bipolar, or manic-depressive, disorder)
- Heavy drinking makes your depression worse

How Serious Is Your Depression?

As important as identifying the cause of your depression is determining the depth of your feelings. If you often have suicidal thoughts, please confide in your physician and a close friend or relative. You will recover, but in your present state you need the support of someone you trust. Share this information and together do the detective work needed to discover what is responsible for your continued depression.

The Seven Kinds of Alcoholic Depression

As I noted earlier, at HRC we have identified seven sources of biochemical depression affecting alcoholics:

1. Neurotransmitter depletion
2. Unavailability of prostaglandin E_1
3. Vitamin/mineral deficiency
4. Hypothyroidism
5. Hypoglycemia
6. Food and chemical allergies
7. Candida-related complex

Where do you fit in? Let's begin with the most likely biochemical scenario.

Neurotransmitter Depletion and Depression

In earlier chapters you became acquainted with neurotransmitters, the natural chemicals that facilitate communication between brain cells. These substances govern our emotions, memory, moods, behavior, sleep, and learning abilities. Neurotransmitters are manufactured in the brain from the amino acids we extract from foods, and their supply is entirely dependent on the presence of these precursor amino acids.

Alcohol destroys these essential precursor amino acids which is probably why alcoholics seem so emotionally muddled and depressed. Without adequate amino-acid conversion, neurotransmitters are no longer produced in sufficient amounts; this deficiency causes "emotional" symptoms, including depression.

The two major neurotransmitters involved in preventing depression are serotonin (converted from the amino acid L-tryptophan) and norepinephrine (converted from the amino acids L-phenylalanine and L-tyrosine). You can resupply these vital neurotransmitters and reverse depression by taking daily amino-acid supplements.

Your symptoms will determine which amino acid you will take for depression: tryptophan if your symptoms are sleeplessness, anxiety, or irritability; L-tyrosine or L-phenylalanine if your symptoms are lethargy, fatigue, sleeping too much, or feelings of immobility.

Tryptophan to Serotonin

The amino acid tryptophan found in large amounts in milk and turkey is the nutrient needed to form serotonin, which controls moods, sleep, sex drive, appetite, and pain threshold. Eating disorders and violent behavior have also been traced to serotonin depletion. Replacing serotonin can lift depression and end insomnia. In one notable study, a medical researcher in Holland demonstrated that a combination of tryptophan (2 grams nightly) and vitamin B_6 (125 milligrams three times a day) could restore patients with anxiety-type depression to normal in four weeks. Depression accompanied by anxiety and sleep disturbances is most likely to respond to tryptophan.

How to Take Tryptophan:

Until the U.S. Food and Drug Administration prohibited the manufacture and sale of tryptophan in the United States in the fall of 1989, we used it for ten years at HRC without any ill effects. This amino acid has also been widely used in England and Canada. Last year, however, a number of deaths and illnesses in the United States were traced to batches of tryptophan manufactured in Japan. In response, the FDA removed tryptophan from the U.S. market. At the time of this writing, the ban remains in effect. I want to caution you against using any tryptophan purchased before the FDA barred its sale. I am confident that eventually tryptophan will again be freely available in this country. At that point, you can purchase a fresh supply. Here are guidelines for its use:

- Tryptophan alone will not be converted to serotonin. To insure that it is properly used, you must also take vitamin C and vitamin B_6 (Table 25).
- Tryptophan is converted to niacin before its final conversion into serotonin. If your body is deficient in niacin, the tryptophan you take will supply you with niacin, not serotonin. For this reason, it is a good idea to take a B-complex vitamin daily. This will give you both vitamin B_6 and niacin and allow the tryptophan to be converted to serotonin.

Of all the amino acids, tryptophan is least able to cross the blood-brain barrier. It must pass this biological hurdle in order to be converted to serotonin. You can give it a nudge by taking it in fruit juice with a half-teaspoon of sugar. This will trigger insulin release, which will assist the tryptophan across the blood-brain barrier. Always take your tryptophan on an empty stomach.

Safety and Side Effects:

Orthomolecular physicians have safely used tryptophan in doses of one to six grams daily. Since it is not stored in the body, it cannot accumulate to toxic levels. However, taking high levels of tryptophan can produce some side effects:

Table 25. The HRC Formula for Depression Due to Serotonin Depletion

Nutrient	Dose	Directions
L-Tryptophan*†	500 mg	2 to 8 capsules per day in divided doses (1 or 2 midmorning, 1 or 2 midafternoon, 2 to 4 at bedtime) on an empty stomach
Vitamin B_6*	50 mg	1 capsule 3 times per day
Vitamin C*	1,000 mg	1 capsule per day
Niacin or Niacinamide (non-time-released)*	500 mg	1 capsule per day

*This level was partly or completely established in your adjusted nutrient plan or in other formulas you may be taking. Refer to your nutrient replacement list (Chart 6 or 7) to determine whether you need to add more of this nutrient to achieve the level suggested here.
†Use tryptophan only if the FDA lifts the current ban on its sale.

- Drowsiness the next morning
- Bizarre or strange dreams (rare)
- Increased blood pressure in persons over age sixty who already have high blood pressure
- Aggressiveness (this rare side effect can occur in the absence of sufficient supplies of the nutrients needed for normal conversion of tryptophan to serotonin)

Who Should Not Take Tryptophan:

- Anyone who takes an MAO (monoamine oxidase) inhibitor for depression; do not take tryptophan until ten days after giving up MAO inhibitors
- Anyone with severe liver disease (a damaged liver cannot properly metabolize tryptophan or any other amino acid)
- Pregnant women (you may be able to take five hundred to a

thousand milligrams of tryptophan, but only with the approval and supervision of your physician)

Tyrosine to Norepinephrine

The amino acid tyrosine, found in large amounts in meats and cheeses, has an amazing effect on depression. A number of studies have found that it can succeed where antidepressant drugs fail.

In the brain, tyrosine is converted into the neurotransmitter norepinephrine, which has been described as the brain's version of adrenaline. You can appreciate the power of norepinephrine when you realize that the high produced by cocaine comes from the drug's ability to activate norepinephrine while inhibiting serotonin. This chemical reaction causes the brain to race until the supply of norepinephrine is depleted. The crash leaves addicts exhausted, depressed, extremely irritable, and craving more cocaine. Large doses of tyrosine can reduce withdrawal symptoms and prevent serious depression among cocaine addicts.

We have used tyrosine at the Health Recovery Center for the past few years with no adverse effects. The usual dose is three to six grams per day, taken on an empty stomach. You must take vitamins B_6 and C to facilitate conversion of tyrosine to norepinephrine (Table 26).

L-Phenylalanine to Norepinephrine

As an alternative to tyrosine, you can take the amino acid L-phenylalanine, which also can be converted into norepinephrine. A number of studies have confirmed L-phenylalanine's amazing antidepressant effects. In one, this potent amino acid was found as effective an antidepressant as the drug imipramine (Tofranil).

L-Phenylalanine has one important advantage over tyrosine in treating depression. It can be converted to a substance called 2-phenylethylamine, or 2-PEA. Low brain levels of 2-PEA are responsible for some depression (before it converts to tyrosine, which then converts to norepinephrine).

If you are affected, L-phenylalanine will be better for you than tyrosine. The only way to find out is by trial and error. I recommend that you start by taking L-phenylalanine. If you find that it makes your

Table 26. The HRC Formula for Depression Due to Norepinephrine Depletion

Nutrient	Dose	Directions
L-Tyrosine	500 mg	4 to 10 capsules per day in 2 or 3 equal doses on an empty stomach
OR		
L-Phenylalanine*	500 mg	1 to 3 capsules per day in equal doses on an empty stomach
Vitamin B_6*	50 mg	1 capsule 3 times per day
Vitamin C*	1,000 mg	1 capsule per day

*This level was partly or completely established in your adjusted nutrient plan or in other formulas you may be taking. Refer to your nutrient replacement list (Chart 6 or 7) to determine whether you need to add more of this nutrient to achieve the level suggested here.

thoughts rush (an effect that is often described as the brain "racing"), you don't need 2-PEA and should switch to tyrosine. The only other disadvantage to taking L-phenylalanine is its slight potential for raising blood pressure. There is also some evidence that excess L-phenylalanine can cause headaches, insomnia, and irritability. For these reasons, it is important to start with a low dose.

L-Phenylalanine doses can range from 500 milligrams to 1,500 milligrams daily taken on an empty stomach. Overdose symptoms are headaches, insomnia, and irritability.

Who Should Not Take Tyrosine or L-Phenylalanine:

- Anyone with high blood pressure should avoid phenylalanine or take very low doses (one hundred milligrams) at first and monitor blood pressure as dosage is increased
- No one taking an MAO inhibitor for depression should take either tyrosine or L-phenylalanine
- No one with severe liver damage should take any amino acid

- Do not take any amino acids during pregnancy except with the approval and supervision of your physician
- No one with PKU (phenylketonuria) should use L-phenylalanine
- No one with schizophrenia should take either amino acid (except with a physician's approval and under his or her supervision)
- No one with an overactive thyroid or malignant melanoma should take either amino acid
- If you are being treated for any serious illness, consult your doctor before taking these amino acids

Unavailability of Prostaglandin E₁ and Depression

Another biochemical cause of depression is a genetic inability to manufacture enough prostaglandin E_1 (PGE_1), an important brain metabolite derived from essential fatty acids. The problem is the result of an inborn deficiency in omega-6 essential fatty acid (EFA). Alcohol stimulates temporary production of PGE_1 and lifts the depression. If you have been depressed since childhood, your introduction to alcohol was probably nothing short of miraculous. But this relief is short-lived. When you stop drinking, PGE_1 levels fall again and depression returns. To banish it, you turn again to alcohol. Thus a deadly spiral begins toward alcoholism. During the last fifteen years, researchers have learned to restore normal PGE_1 levels in alcoholics and eliminate both the depression and the need to drink for relief. A substance called gamma-linolenic acid (GLA) is easily converted to PGE_1. I have seen some amazing recoveries from depression within three weeks of GLA treatment.

Take the case of Colleen, a high school English teacher. Colleen described her childhood and teenage years as withdrawn and lonely. "I can't remember not being depressed," she told me. In college, she drank alcohol for the first time and received the shock of her young life. Her world brightened in a way she had never before experienced. She felt different. Friendly. Happy. The effects lingered into the next day, and then gloom closed in again. After experiencing the dramatic lift in her spirits, she was convinced that she had discovered a magic elixir in alcohol. In a short time she was drinking a few beers every day. The alcohol never failed to banish her depression.

As her college years passed, Colleen's alcohol consumption escalated. She needed to drink more and more to get the lift she sought. She also began to experience deep depressions in the days following heavy drinking. After college, she began teaching high school English. Controlling her depression with alcohol became a real balancing act. Eventually, her drinking came to the attention of her peers and her students. Colleen was appalled at the idea that she was a problem drinker. She decided to prove she could live without alcohol.

The next ten years were some of the most miserable of her life. She joined AA and sought psychiatric help for her severe depression. Sadly, no antidepressant drug relieved her misery. It was hard to keep teaching, hard to keep living. Her depression had reached the suicidal stage when she reasoned that alcohol could put an end to her despair. Her decision to resume drinking didn't take much reflection. Predictably, her alcohol intake began to escalate rapidly. This time, no one sympathized. Her principal ordered her to treatment. Three weeks after completing an inpatient program, she was back at work and drinking again to medicate her depression. A second round of treatment left her temporarily dry and depressed. Colleen was on a merry-go-round she couldn't get off. When she called the Health Recovery Center, she was crying: "I have alienated everyone because I won't stay sober, but being drunk feels better than being depressed."

I often think someone up there does watch over people; it seems more than coincidence that Colleen found her way to one of the only treatment centers in the country that would run tests and restore her chemistry to normal. Within three weeks, her depression had vanished. She no longer needed nor craved alcohol.

Colleen's was a classic case of chronic depression caused by too little PGE_1. Although alcohol blocks production of additional amounts of this metabolite, its active effect is to enhance what little is available in the brain. Eventually, a no-win situation develops and alcohol becomes the only way to prevent depression. The solution, of course, is to provide the brain with the PGE_1 needed to reverse the depression. Figure 9 shows how essential fatty acids are converted into PGE_1 and other brain metabolites. If your body can't do this normally, you can correct the problem by taking gamma-linolenic acid (GLA) in the form of Efamol (a trade name for oil of evening primrose). The formula for EFA deficient depression (Table 27) includes three supportive nutri-

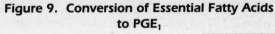

**Figure 9. Conversion of Essential Fatty Acids
to PGE₁**

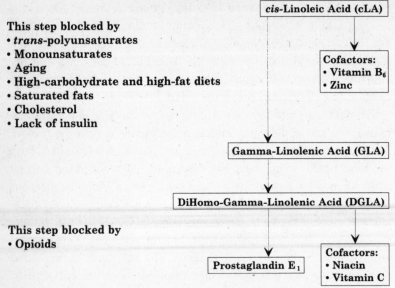

cis-Linoleic Acid (cLA)

This step blocked by
• trans-polyunsaturates
• Monounsaturates
• Aging
• High-carbohydrate and high-fat diets
• Saturated fats
• Cholesterol
• Lack of insulin

Cofactors:
• Vitamin B₆
• Zinc

Gamma-Linolenic Acid (GLA)

DiHomo-Gamma-Linolenic Acid (DGLA)

This step blocked by
• Opioids

Prostaglandin E₁

Cofactors:
• Niacin
• Vitamin C

From D. Horrobin et al., "Possible Role of Prostaglandin E₁ in Affective Disorders and in Alcoholism," British Medical Journal 1 (June 1980): 1363–66.

ents in addition to Efamol: zinc, needed for formation of gamma-linolenic acid (GLA); vitamin B₆, for metabolism of *cis*-linoleic acid; and vitamin C, to increase production of PGE₁. When you take GLA and its cofactors, depression magically lifts and won't return as long as you continue to take the formula. Colleen now uses this natural substance daily instead of alcohol, and her world has brightened up permanently.

Do You Have an EFA Deficiency?

In his book *Essential Fatty Acids and Immunity in Mental Health,* Charles Bates, Ph.D., provides a list of factors that suggest an essential fatty acid deficiency:

• Ancestry that is one-quarter or more Celtic Irish, Scandinavian, native American, Welsh, or Scottish

Table 27. The HRC Formula for Depression due to EFA Deficiency

Nutrient	Dose	Directions
Efamol*	500 mg	3 capsules 3 times per day with meals (9 per day); can be reduced to 6 per day after 1 month
Zinc picolinate*	20 mg	1 capsule with food
Vitamin B_6*	50 mg	1 capsule 3 times per day
Vitamin C*	1,000 mg	1 capsule per day
Niacin	100 mg	1 capsule with food daily

*This level was partly or completely established in your adjusted nutrient plan or in other formulas you may be taking. Refer to your nutrient replacement list (Chart 6 or 7) to determine whether you need to add more of this nutrient to achieve the level suggested here.

- A tendency to abuse alcohol or feel that it affects you differently from others; trouble with alcohol in your teenage years
- Anxiety or depression during hangovers
- Depression among close relatives
- A family history of alcoholism, depression, suicide, schizophrenia, or other mental illness, religious fanaticism, or fanatical teetotaling
- Depression that persists while you are abstinent from alcohol
- A personal or family history of Crohn's disease, hepatic cirrhosis, cystic fibrosis, Sjögren-Larsson syndrome, atopic eczema
- A personal or family history of ulcerative colitis, irritable bowel syndrome, premenstrual syndrome, scleroderma, diabetes, or benign breast disease
- Experiencing an emotional lift from certain foods or vitamins
- Winter depressions that lighten in the spring

Vitamin and Mineral Deficiency and Depression

The effect of nutritional deficiencies on brain chemistry can cause depression, anger, listlessness, and paranoia. Unfortunately, the connection between depression and vitamin and mineral deficiencies is often missed. At Johns Hopkins University, sixty-nine cases of scurvy (total vitamin C depletion) were discovered at autopsy, and yet the disease had not been diagnosed before death in 91 percent of these patients.

One of the most dramatic cases of vitamin and mineral deficiencies I have seen involved a man I'll call Paul. He had been arrested four times for drunken driving but continued to drink daily. His probation officer brought him to the Health Recovery Center. The three of us had to decide if an outpatient program would be proper for someone as depressed as Paul. The court had just ordered him back to treatment; judging by the miserable look on his face, it was the last place he wanted to be.

Paul was thirty, divorced and living alone. He rarely ate more than one meal a day, usually fast food or junk food. He lived on coffee, cigarettes, and beer. Paul confided that he was probably going to lose his sales job because he could no longer motivate himself. He blamed all of his troubles on depression. There were so many aspects of his life-style that suggested a real depletion of the natural chemicals he needed to recover from alcoholism and depression that I urged Paul to let us work with him.

Two days later, after receiving his B-complex shots, Paul remarked that we must have injected him with an amphetamine. The effect of restoring these life-giving substances was dramatic. He also made many life-style changes that contributed to his recovery, but one of the most important was the replacement of certain key natural substances that helped relieve his depression.

The B-Complex Vitamins

The B-complex vitamins are essential to mental and emotional well-being. They cannot be stored in our bodies, so we depend entirely on our daily diet to supply them. B vitamins are destroyed by alcohol, refined sugars, nicotine, and caffeine—the very substances that most alcoholics consume almost to the exclusion of everything else. Small wonder that deficiences develop. Here's a rundown of recent finding about the relationship of B-complex vitamins to depression:

- Vitamin B_1 (thiamine): Deficiencies trigger depression and irritability and can cause neurological and cardiac disorders among alcoholics.
- Vitamin B_2 (riboflavin): In 1982 an article published in the *British Journal of Psychiatry* reported that every one of 172 successive patients admitted to a British psychiatric hospital for treatment of depression was deficient in B_2.
- Vitamin B_3 (niacin): Depletion causes anxiety, depression, apprehension, and fatigue.
- Vitamin B_5 (pantothenic acid): Symptoms of deficiency are fatigue, chronic stress, and depression. Vitamin B_5 is needed for hormone formation and the uptake of amino acids and the brain chemical acetylcholine, which combine to prevent certain types of depression.
- Vitamin B_6 (pyridoxine): Deficiency can disrupt formation of neurotransmitters. Vitamin B_6 is a coenzyme needed for conversion of tryptophan to serotonin and phenylalanine and tyrosine to norepinephrine. I have discussed the relationships of these neurotransmitters to depression earlier in this chapter.
- Vitamin B_{12}: Deficiency will cause depression.
- Folic acid: Deficiency is a common cause of depression.

Vitamin C

Continuing vitamin C deficiency causes chronic depression, fatigue, and vague ill health.

Minerals

Deficiencies in a number of minerals can also cause depression. If this is at the root of your problem, you should already be on the road to recovery; your adjusted nutrient plan contains sufficient amounts of all the minerals necessary to overcome any deficiencies. But I would like you to familiarize yourself with the minerals that can underlie depression so you can better understand the rationale for taking large doses of so many supplements.

- Magnesium: Symptoms of deficiency include confusion, apathy, loss of appetite, weakness, and insomnia.
- Calcium: Depletion affects the central nervous system. Low levels of calcium cause nervousness, apprehension, irritability, and numbness.
- Zinc: Inadequacies result in apathy, lack of appetite, and lethargy. When zinc is low, copper in the body can increase to toxic levels, resulting in paranoia and fearfulness.
- Iron: Depression is often a symptom of chronic iron deficiency. Other symptoms include general weakness, listlessness, exhaustion, lack of appetite, and headaches.
- Manganese: This metal is needed for proper use of the B-complex vitamins and vitamin C. Since it also plays a role in amino-acid formation, a deficiency may contribute to depression stemming from low levels of the neurotransmitters serotonin and norepinephrine. Manganese also helps stabilize blood sugar and prevent hypoglycemic mood swings.
- Potassium: Depletion is frequently associated with depression, tearfulness, weakness, and fatigue. A 1981 study found that depressed patients were more likely than controls to have decreased intracellular potassium. Decreased brain levels of potassium have also been found on autopsy of suicides. You can boost your potassium intake by using one teaspoon of Morton's Lite-Salt every day.

The Safety of Supplements

Vitamin C and the B-complex vitamins discussed above are all water soluble. This means that they can't accumulate in your body or be stored for future use. Amounts above and beyond your current nutritional needs are dumped into your urine. As a result, there is no danger of overdose.

Unlike water soluble vitamins, minerals can be stored in your tissues. Refer to Table 24 for the RDAs and therapeutic treatment levels. Do not exceed the recommended therapeutic doses, since accumulation of minerals in the body can be dangerous.

Hypothyroidism and Depression

The stress showed on Mary's face as she described how weary and depressed she felt. Her husband and children demanded too much of her, and she drank to escape the pressures and responsibilities. Mary had been in our program for two weeks. She was now alcohol free and making life-style changes. Still, she had very little energy and didn't seem to be recovering very fast.

As we talked, she inadvertently offered several clues to the source of her problem. She complained that even on her restricted diet she simply couldn't lose weight. Exercise was out of the question. She was just too tired, even though she slept up to ten hours a night. She was wearing a heavy sweater even though it was a warm spring day. She said she had a hard time keeping warm and was very susceptible to catching colds. By the end of our session, I had heard enough to refer her to our physician for a thyroid test.

Symptoms of hypothyroidism (low thyroid function) include

- Depression
- Mental sluggishness
- Confusion
- Poor memory
- Fatigue
- Low sex drive
- Brittle hair
- Dry skin
- Puffiness around the eyes
- Cold hands and feet
- Sleeping more than eight hours a night
- Susceptibility to colds and infections

Researchers speculate that hypothyroidism causes depression because there is an insufficient supply of oxygen to the brain, since people with low thyroid function do not use oxygen efficiently. Linus Pauling contends that all depression could be eliminated if brain cells received sufficient oxygen.

Testing

If you have any of the symptoms listed above, you can test yourself for hypothyroidism with a procedure first described in the *Journal of the American Medical Association* by thyroid expert Broda Barnes, M.D. The test could not be simpler. People with low thyroid function have lower than normal body temperatures because they are not burning up as much food as they should. All you have to do for this test is determine whether your body temperature is lower than normal.

Use a digital or basal thermometer, not a fever thermometer. The basal type is commonly used by women trying to get pregnant—or trying to avoid pregnancy—to determine when ovulation occurs on the basis of an increase in body temperature. Basal thermometers are available in most drugstores.

Upon waking, place the thermometer snugly under your armpit for ten minutes. If it registers below 97.8 degrees *and* if you have symptoms of hypothyroidism, you probably need thyroid hormone.

This home test can give you a fix on your thyroid status. If you haven't yet been tested, you can ask your doctor to check further. The usual laboratory tests for thyroid (T_3, T_4, and TSH) do not always tell the whole story. But a new test, the fluorescence activated microsphere assay (available from ImmunoDiagnostic Laboratories in San Leandro, California) will often reveal abnormalities less sophisticated tests miss.

In Mary's case, standard lab tests indicated low-normal thyroid function, but her morning temperature never rose above 96.9 degrees. We treated her with Armour Thyroid, a prescription drug. It relieved her depression and eliminated her mental sluggishness and fatigue. She also lost weight.

If your home thyroid test shows that your temperature is consistently below 97.8 degrees, see your physician to discuss treatment. If the doctor wants more information on your testing method, refer him or her to Dr. Barnes's book *Hypothyroidism: The Unsuspected Illness*. Another useful book is *Solving the Puzzle of Illness* by Steven Langer, M.D.

Dr. Barnes has published more than a hundred papers and several books on the role of the thyroid gland in human health. He treats thyroid disorders with natural desiccated thyroid (bovine or pork) rather than synthetic thyroid preparations. The advantage of natural thyroid over synthetic is that all thyroid hormones are replaced with the natural product, whereas synthetics have not yet been able to duplicate nature completely and do not affect two troublesome symptoms of hypothyroidism, dry skin and water retention.

Hypoglycemia and Depression

In his studies of twelve hundred hypoglycemic patients, Stephen Gyland, M.D., found that 86 percent were depressed. More recently, positron emission tomography (PET) scans have verified that glucose metabolism is often reduced in the brains of patients suffering from depression.

Table 28, which is based on Dr. Gyland's work, compares the symptoms of hypoglycemia and depression. It is no accident that both conditions are so common among alcoholics. If hypoglycemia underlies your depression, you should begin to notice an improvement soon after you adopt the hypoglycemic diet recommended in Chapter 7.

Food and Chemical Allergies and Depression

The connection between food allergies and depression was a revelation to me. I was treating a young woman who was both alcoholic and depressed. I expected to find some food or chemical sensitivities because she had a terrible withdrawal hangover when she stopped drinking, indicating an allergic/addicted response to alcohol. But I was not prepared for the Jekyll and Hyde changes that I witnessed. By the end of a week-long modified fast, Carol was feeling much better. Her depression was gone, and her energy had returned. Then she tested wheat. Within two hours she crashed. Crying over the telephone, she told me she was too depressed to continue the program. The next day she apologized. We were both grateful to find a major trigger to her depression.

Table 28. Symptoms of Hypoglycemia and Depression

Hypoglycemia	Depression
Nervousness	Nervousness
Irritability	Irritability
Exhaustion	Exhaustion
Faintness, cold sweats	—
Depression	Depression
Drowsiness	Drowsiness
Insomnia	Insomnia
Constant worrying	Constant worrying
Mental confusion	Mental confusion
Rapid pulse	Rapid pulse
Internal trembling	Internal trembling
Forgetfulness	Forgetfulness
Headache	Headache
Unprovoked anxieties	Unprovoked anxieties
Digestive disturbances	—

After her severe reaction, I expected Carol to avoid wheat religiously. At the time, I didn't understand the addiction aspect of the allergic/addicted response. Carol had enormous cravings for breads and pasta, so her resolve lasted only a few days. Then she succumbed to temptation and ate pizza for lunch. An hour later, she arrived at her treatment group sobbing inconsolably while the others groped for emotional explanations for her behavior. After her wheat reaction wore off, her depression again lifted.

Wheat is not the only substance capable of triggering a maladaptive reaction within the brains and nervous systems of sensitive people. Alcohol, certain foods (particularly the grains from which alcohol is made), and many chemicals (particularly hydrocarbon-based products like gasoline and paints) can also cause reactions. Food addiction keeps us coming back for more of certain foods. We love the initial mild highs they provide as they lift us out of our withdrawal state. We don't understand that the downside of this addiction is depression, anxiety, and mental confusion, the result of the inevitable withdrawal in the nervous system and the brain.

If you are an allergic/addicted alcoholic, consider the possibility that substances other than alcohol may be affecting your brain and causing depression. In Chapter 11 you'll learn how to identify and eliminate these culprits.

Candida-Related Complex and Depression

During the last five years, we have seen a steady parade of clients who are fighting an internal war with an overgrowth of a common intestinal yeast called *Candida albicans*. I can usually tell on the basis of a first interview who is a probable candidate for treatment of candida-related complex (CRC). People suffering from this problem appear depressed, tired, anxious, and so spacey that they can't follow what I'm saying. They tell me they continually crave sugar as well as alcohol, and they have telltale signs of yeast invasion throughout their bodies. Their immune systems are so depressed that most foods cause bloating and produce allergic/addictive responses. If you suffer from CRC, your depression won't lift until these yeast colonizers are brought under control.

In Chapter 11 you'll find a full discussion of CRC and its symptoms, as well as an explanation for why some people are particularly susceptible to this yeast. There is also a description of the tests and treatment for CRC.

Suicide and Depression

Before we leave the subject of depression, I want to discuss a painful subject: suicide, the final solution to depression. If your life, like mine, has been seared by the suicide of a family member, you may find the answers you have been seeking. And if you have been trying to cope with overwhelming depression and are plagued with thoughts of suicide, you will find a welcome warning that can help you avert tragedy.

Over the years, I've learned that alcoholics often conceal the fact that family members have taken their own lives. But if I tell them about my son's suicide, the truth comes rushing out: "My father shot himself" or "Several times, my mother took a deliberate overdose of pills" or "My son hung himself." The pain of these tragic deaths is often compounded by a family code of silence. Often, those touched by the tragedy are tormented by guilt. They can't stop wondering whether they could have done anything to prevent the suicide, whether they missed warning signs that tragedy was approaching. Recent scientific findings provide some of the answers to these agonizing questions and offer comfort and insight.

Most people experience some major disappointment or stress in the course of life, but suicide is rarely the outcome. And, there is no good evidence suggesting that most depression predates alcoholism or that any personality traits underlie alcoholism. Indeed, researchers have so far failed to find genetically transmitted depression among most alcoholics. Instead, studies suggest that the prolonged use of alcohol causes biochemical changes in the brain associated with depression and suicide. The most striking of these findings (from the National Institute of Mental Health) shows that the neurotransmitter serotonin is almost depleted in all the brains of suicides examined during autopsies. Since alcoholism causes the destruction of tryptophan and other precursor amino acids needed for production of the antidepressant neurotransmitters, it's not surprising that many alcoholics are prone to depression and even suicide. As I have explained earlier in this chapter, alcohol can also precipitate depression by destroying a number of other natural chemicals, including

- The neurotransmitter norepinephrine, formed from the amino acids phenylalanine and tyrosine
- Endorphins
- Essential fatty acids needed to form brain metabolites, including prostaglandin E_1 (PGE_1)
- B vitamins, which supply the brain's energy and maintain mental and emotional balance

- Trace elements and enzymes that govern the body's hormonal balance

A cerebral allergic reaction to alcohol or other substances can cause suicidal depression. You'll find a full discussion of this effect in Chapter 11. High levels of toxins from *Candida albicans* overgrowth can also affect the brain and central nervous system and induce suicidal depression. Alcoholism promotes both proliferation of candida and escalation of cerebral allergies.

Since alcohol can inflict so much biochemical damage on the brain and nervous system, it should not be surprising that many alcoholics attempt suicide. One recent study found that up to 40 percent of all alcoholics try to take their own lives at least once; another study found that 25 percent of the deaths of treated alcoholics were suicides.

If you feel that you or someone close to you is a suicide risk, please reread this chapter carefully and make the changes recommended to restore normal balance and banish depression once and for all.

Where Do You Fit In?

Now that you are familiar with the various problems that can underlie depression, it's time to determine what to do about the one(s) responsible for your own bleak state of mind. Here are the options. Check all the categories that apply to you:

_____ Restoring the neurotransmitters serotonin and/or norepinephrine (formulas in this chapter)

_____ Replacing essential fatty acids to create PGE_1 (formula in this chapter)

_____ Restoring key vitamins and minerals (review the list of vitamins and minerals earlier in this chapter)

_____ Treating hypothyroidism (consult your physician)

_____ Correcting hypoglycemia (review Chapter 7)

_____ Avoiding foods/chemicals responsible for cerebral allergy/addiction (see Chapter 11)

_____ Treating candida-related complex (see Chapter 11)

Don't be surprised if you fit several of these seven categories. Heavy alcohol use wreaks havoc on your biochemical balance. But with the HRC repair program you can restore your health. In some cases you'll need a physician's help. I can't overemphasize the importance of expert medical advice when you are dealing with depression, especially if it is severe. It is equally important to choose a doctor attuned to your special needs.

Orthomolecular MDs are experts in both allopathic and nutritional science who treat disorders at the cellular level with biological weapons—nutrients that nature has provided in her own system of defense for millions of years. An orthomolecular psychiatrist or physician can help you address the following problems:

- Restoration of neurotransmitter levels via amino-acid therapy
- Hypoglycemia testing and treatment
- Vitamin, mineral, and essential fatty acid testing and restoration
- Thyroid testing and treatment

For a list of orthomolecular physicians in your area, contact the Huxley Institute for Biosocial Research, 900 North Federal Highway, Boca Raton, FL 33432, (800) 847-3802.

A clinical ecologist will be able to test you for food and chemical allergies and candida-related complex. For a list of such physicians in your area, contact the American Academy of Environmental Medicine, P.O. Box 16106, Denver, CO 80216, (303) 622-9755.

Eleven

Week Six: Biochemical Traps That Block Recovery

If you have been faithfully following the biochemical repair program outlined so far and still do not feel as well as you suspect you should, you may be wondering whether this program is right for you. Relax. This program *will* work for all alcoholics, but you may be suffering from food allergies or chemical sensitivities that must be identified and treated before your recovery can be complete. Or you may be battling an overgrowth of *Candida albicans,* a yeast that can sap your energy and undermine your health. Alcoholics are particularly vulnerable to candida overgrowth. In this chapter, I'll discuss each of these complex conditions. You'll learn how to determine whether you are affected and, if so, what you can do to overcome these debilitating disorders. I have seen some dramatic recoveries among clients who discover that they are afflicted with one or more of these problems.

Chemical Sensitivities

When I suspect that a client is chemically sensitive, I always tell the story of Roger, a counselor at an alcoholism detox center who had not had a drink since he had completed traditional treatment three years before I met him. Underneath the veneer of success, Roger was tormented by explosive anger, anxiety, and exhaustion. When he called me, he said his dry-drunk behavior was threatening his job. He didn't know how to control his emotions and was afraid that he would wind up drinking again. Worse, he recognized that he was having suicidal thoughts. He was very frightened.

At our initial interview, I discovered that Roger was consuming twenty-five cups of coffee and a six-pack of cola every day. Correcting his hypoglycemia soon calmed the mood swings, but his behavior was still unpredictable. Not until he told me about his hobby, taxidermy, did I begin to suspect the culprit. In his off-hours, Roger was inhaling solvents, glues, and thinners that just might explain the symptoms that continued to trouble him. To find out, I sent him to a clinical ecologist for tests. His reaction to ethanols and formaldehydes was dramatic. Upon exposure in the lab, he became quite anxious and paranoid. Tests also revealed sensitivities to wheat and dairy products that brought on delayed reactions of severe irritability and fatigue.

When Roger was drinking, withdrawal from alcohol typically brought on violent scenes and bleak moods. Although he had managed to quit, for permanent relief he had to avoid the other substances that altered his brain chemistry and undermined his emotional stability. Roger recovered by giving up caffeine, nicotine, refined sugars, wheat, and dairy products and minimizing his exposure to ethanols and formaldehyde.

Over the years I have learned that house painters, garage mechanics, hair stylists, printers, and others who continually breathe chemical fumes on the job are often alcoholic. At the end of the workday they are literally intoxicated by the fumes from their jobs, and they head straight to the bar to forestall withdrawal symptoms. Those who try to stop drinking develop unrelenting cravings for alcohol.

A distinguished Chicago allergist, Theron Randolph, M.D., was the first to propose that many physical and emotional disorders may be related to exposure to environmental chemicals. He discovered that susceptible people first experience a pleasing, addictive high followed eventually by withdrawal symptoms. Figure 10, adapted from Randolph's book *An Alternative Approach to Allergies,* will give you an idea of the range of these symptoms from the initial "up" to the subsequent withdrawal or "down." The more you are stimulated (intoxicated) by the chemical, the more severe the withdrawal will be.

A Health Recovery Center study showed that 56 percent of our clients were sensitive to chemicals in the environment. The most common offender was ethanol, contained in a wide range of products, including

- Natural gas
- Gasoline (regular and diesel)
- Some paints
- Automobile exhaust
- Alcohols

Figure 10. The Ups and Downs of Addiction

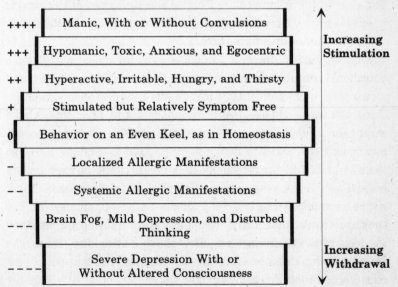

++++	Manic, With or Without Convulsions
+++	Hypomanic, Toxic, Anxious, and Egocentric
++	Hyperactive, Irritable, Hungry, and Thirsty
+	Stimulated but Relatively Symptom Free
0	Behavior on an Even Keel, as in Homeostasis
_	Localized Allergic Manifestations
_ _	Systemic Allergic Manifestations
_ _ _	Brain Fog, Mild Depression, and Disturbed Thinking
_ _ _ _	Severe Depression With or Without Altered Consciousness

Increasing Stimulation

Increasing Withdrawal

- Soft plastics (new car odors)
- Certain hand lotions and perfumes
- Disinfectant cleaners
- Tobacco smoke
- Hydrocarbons

The most common reactions are fatigue, exhaustion, spaciness, mental confusion, depression, cravings, irritability. The magnitude and severity of these responses is startling—sudden intense anger, tears and sobbing, falling asleep, the inability to think or speak coherently.

These symptoms can be readily produced and extinguished in an allergy lab. Testing involves placing a sample of the suspect chemical under the tongue (sublingual testing). If a reaction occurs, it can be turned off by placing a much smaller neutralizing dose of the same substance under the tongue. These test results provide convincing evidence for skeptical clients and those who suspect that their symptoms are all in their minds.

Test Yourself for Chemical Sensitivities

The chemical screening test in Chart 8 was developed at HRC and is based on a questionnaire originally developed by Theron Randolph, M.D., the "father of clinical ecology."

If on the basis of this test you believe you are chemically allergic, you should consult a clinical ecologist/allergist for further testing and treatment. I was tested at Dr. Kroker's office in La Crosse, Wisconsin. The result was a real eye-opener. Before exposure, I had completed a short exercise that required me to match symbols. After the mysterious dose, I was asked to match another page of symbols. I was so sleepy and muddled that I simply could not perform the exercise at a normal pace. I felt as though my IQ had dropped fifty points. Then, with a neutralizing dose under my tongue, I slowly brightened up. The substance responsible for my sleepiness and confusion was ethanol, the base of most perfumes and after-shave lotions. The test results explained why I had been having trouble concentrating when new clients wore a lot of cologne or after-shave.

Chart 8. The Health Recovery Center
Chemical Screening Test

Does exposure to any of the following substances tend to provoke a response from strong dislike to noticeable symptoms?

	Yes	No
1. Newspaper print		
2. Soft plastics (i.e., vinyl, acrylic)		
3. Tobacco smoke		
4. Fabric-store odors		
5. Diesel or auto exhaust		
6. Cooking gas		
7. Pesticide sprays		
8. Insecticide strips		
9. Mothballs or crystals		
10. Fabric softeners (i.e., Bounce)		
11. Detergents		
12. Ammonias		
13. Bleaches		
14. Scented cosmetics		
15. Scented perfumes or after-shaves		
16. Scented deodorants, antiperspirants		
17. Oven cleaner		
18. Furniture polish		
19. Floor wax		
20. New carpets		
21. New car odors		
22. House paints		
23. Turpentines		
24. Foam rubber pillows		
25. Copier machines		

Chart 8. The Health Recovery Center
Chemical Screening Test *(Continued)*

	Yes	No
Answer yes or no to the following questions:		
1. Do you live near heavy traffic?		
2. Do you live near factory pollution?		
3. Do you live near crop spraying?		
4. Do you have a gas clothes dryer?		
5. Do you have a gas water heater?		
6. Do you have a gas kitchen stove?		
7. Do you have a gas fireplace?		
8. Do you have a gas space heater?		
9. Do you feel worse in the winter when your home is more closed up?		
10. Are you aware of smelling any odors upon entering your house? Musty, moldy smells? New house smells? Plastic smells? Leaky gas?		
11. Is your sense of smell below average?		
12. Have you been bothered by chemicals that you encounter on the job?		
13. Have you been exposed to chemicals at work either now or in past jobs?		
14. Do you have hobbies that involve working with glues, solvents, paints, or other chemicals?		
15. Do you classify yourself as an allergic/addicted alcohol biotype?		
TOTAL yes answers		

SCORING: If you are an allergic/addicted alcohol biotype and have fifteen or more yes answers, it is highly likely that you are chemically sensitive.

How to Turn Off Chemical Reactions

Once substances that trigger negative reactions are identified, clinical ecologists can desensitize you with a three-step procedure.

First, they'll prepare a neutralizing dose containing minute amounts of the chemical(s) to which you are sensitive. When this is placed under your tongue, the allergic reaction diminishes within minutes. At the same time, the ability of your immune system to handle the chemical begins to strengthen. You may get a prescription to take home and use according to the doctor's instructions. You may have to use it daily until your immune system can handle exposure normally.

Second, he or she will recommend that you take sodium and potassium bicarbonate in the form of Alka-Seltzer Gold or alkali salts available with a prescription. The salts effectively neutralize the excess acidity that develops in the body during allergic reactions. Two tablets of Alka-Seltzer Gold quickly reduce symptoms that occur after chemical exposure. The adult dose is two tablets every four hours; do not exceed eight tablets in a twenty-four hour period.

Third, to prevent reactions in the future, it is essential that you avoid, as much as possible, the chemicals to which you are sensitive. Also avoid or eliminate chemicals in your home that could potentially cause you problems, including

- Cigarette smoke
- Gas appliances
- Perfumed cosmetics and hair sprays
- Soft vinyl and acrylic items
- Spray cleaners for ovens, baths, and kitchens
- Air fresheners

You can further reduce your exposure by drinking deep well water or bottled spring water instead of chlorinated tap water and avoiding foods that have been heavily sprayed with chemicals (switch to organically grown products). Room and car air filters can also help minimize exposure to chemical fumes. If you must inhale strong chemical odors at work, a portable charcoal mask can help protect you.

Where to Find a Doctor

For a referral to a clinical ecologist in your area who can test and treat you for chemical sensitivities contact the American Academy of Environmental Medicine, P.O. Box 16106, Denver, CO 80216, (303) 622-9755.

Appendix B lists a number of excellent books on chemical hypersensitivity that will give you more information on this common problem.

Food Allergies

The amazing changes that alcohol can trigger in the allergic/addicted alcoholic demonstrate how profoundly the brain is affected by substances it cannot tolerate. Reactions can include anger, loss of control, physical fights, crying, and suicide attempts. If you are allergic/addicted, you may have inherited a biological predisposition to food and chemical intolerances. If so, problems usually begin to develop after you start using the allergenic substance frequently. Your first encounter with it probably made you sick, but with prolonged use your body adapts in a way that suggests you are tolerating the substance. In fact, an addiction is gradually building. When the substance is present, you feel a lift or high. Withdrawal triggers a number of unpleasant or painful symptoms ranging from depression to exhaustion. Unfortunately, giving up alcohol won't necessarily eliminate these problems. Your addictive needs may soon lead you elsewhere for a fix. You may drink pots of coffee laced with sugar or get your high from binging on foods containing the same grains as the alcohol you used to drink. Or you may chain-smoke and drink colas continually. If so, your behavior will be almost as erratic as it was when you were drinking.

Compulsive Eating and Food Allergy

Do you crave certain foods the way drug addicts crave a fix? If so, you may be allergic/addicted to those foods. When this is the case, the foods in question are improperly metabolized in your body and trigger psychoactive chemicals that produce an initial high soon followed by a loss of control (binging) and other negative symptoms like fogginess, fatigue, and depression. Life becomes one binge after another, and weight begins to accumulate. Eventually, some affected individuals turn bulimic to control their weight. The alternative is anorexia nervosa and starvation. If an allergic/addicted person cuts food intake and subsists on salads and vegetables, their cravings will probably subside. This regime eliminates the volatile foods that trigger binges, but it will also deplete stores of the natural chemicals needed for normal brain functioning.

A number of studies have shown that eating disorders like bulimia and anorexia nervosa are linked to zinc deficiencies, possibly because zinc affects our taste, sense of smell, and appetite. In a study at Stanford University, a group of zinc-deficient anorexic adolescents were given supplements, while a control group got none. The youngsters taking zinc began to gain weight. Their senses of taste and smell improved, and their depression and anxious moods lifted. They also began to mature sexually (sexual development can be arrested among anorexic adolescents).

Obesity can also be associated with zinc deficiency. A study at the University of Tennessee Medical Center showed that people who repeatedly regain weight after dieting (victims of the so-called yo-yo syndrome) can lose again without dieting by taking liquid zinc supplements. The Tennessee-study participants lost three to five pounds per month with no other life-style changes.

Are You Allergic to Any Foods?

The self-screening test in Chart 9 designed by George Kroker, M.D., will give you a good idea of foods to which you may be allergic. Follow these instructions:

1. Complete all five parts of the chart
2. In part 5 circle any foods you have listed in part 3
3. (Women only) In part 5 circle any foods you have listed in part 3
4. In part 5 circle any headings that contain foods eaten 6 or 7 days per week

Chart 9. Screening Test for Food Allergies

1. List a typical day's meals and snacks:

Breakfast	Lunch	Dinner	Snacks
_____	_____	_____	_____
_____	_____	_____	_____
_____	_____	_____	_____
_____	_____	_____	_____

2. List your three most favorite foods that you ate regularly before starting this program:

_____   _____   _____

3. Do you crave or binge on any foods? If so, which ones?

_____   _____   _____

_____   _____   _____

4. (For women) Do you crave or binge on foods premenstrually? If so, which ones?

_____   _____   _____

_____   _____   _____

5. Food Questionnaire

How many days in one week do you eat the following foods?
(Write the number of days in the parentheses following the food.)

Wheat

Bread ( )
Rolls ( )
Muffins ( )
Sandwiches ( )
Bagels ( )
Pasta ( )
Macaroni ( )
Noodles ( )
Spaghetti ( )
Casseroles ( )
Pizza ( )
Breakfast Cereal ( )
Crackers ( )
Cookies ( )
Canned Soup ( )
Pastries ( )

Corn

Popcorn ( )
Lunch meat ( )
Corn flakes ( )
Corn (vegetable) ( )
Pancake syrup ( )
Tacos ( )

Other Grains

Rice ( )
Oatmeal ( )
Other:
_____ ( )

Dairy

Milk ( )
Cheese ( )

Yogurt ( )
Ice cream ( )
Coffee creamer ( )
Margarine ( )
Butter ( )
Cream cheese ( )
Cottage cheese ( )

Eggs

Scrambled,
  omelet, etc. ( )
Mayonnaise ( )
French toast ( )

Yeast

Mushrooms ( )
Vinegar ( )
Salad dressing ( )
Soy sauce ( )
Raisins ( )
Dates ( )
Prunes ( )
Ketchup ( )
Mustard ( )
Fruit juice ( )

Snacks/Miscellaneous

Potato chips ( )
Chocolate ( )
Peanuts ( )
Other nuts:
_____ ( )
Dessert:
_____ ( )
Jell-O ( )

Jelly/jam ( )
Sweet 'N Low ( )
Equal ( )

Beef

Hamburger ( )
Steak ( )
Beef roast ( )

Pork

Ham ( )
Bacon ( )
Sausage ( )
Pork chops ( )

Other Protein

Chicken ( )
Turkey ( )
Fish:
_____ ( )
_____ ( )
Soy/tofu ( )
Hot dogs ( )

Beverages

Coffee ( )
Tea ( )
Soda: ( )
_____ ( )
Diet soda: ( )
_____ ( )
Alcoholic
  beverages:
_____ ( )

Chart 9. Screening Test for Food Allergies (*Continued*)

Fruit		Potatoes/		Spices		
		french fries	( )			
Apples	( )	Tomato	( )	Onion	( )	
Bananas	( )	Green pepper	( )	Garlic	( )	
Oranges	( )	Peas	( )	Pepper	( )	
Pears	( )	Green beans	( )	Dry mustard	( )	
Melon	( )	Other beans:		Basil	( )	
Grapefruit	( )			Paprika	( )	
Grapes	( )	_____	( )	Rosemary	( )	
Pineapple	( )	Carrots	( )	Ginger	( )	
Other:		Celery	( )	Parsley	( )	
_____	( )	Broccoli	( )	Oregano	( )	
_____	( )	Cabbage/		Cinnamon	( )	
		coleslaw	( )	Mint	( )	
		Cauliflower	( )	Other:		
		Other:				
Vegetables		_____	( )	_____	( )	
Lettuce salads	( )	_____	( )			

The foods you identify are the ones most likely to trigger addictive cravings and delayed allergic reactions.

You can get expert medical help with diagnosing and treating food allergies by contacting a physician who specializes in clinical ecology. For a list of qualified physicians in your area, write or call the American Academy of Environmental Mecicine, P.O. Box 16106, Denver, CO 80216, (303) 622-9755.

You can take some steps to control food allergies on your own. Remove the suspected foods from your diet, don't buy them when you shop, and remove them from your cupboards and refrigerator. Replace them with foods you don't often eat.

For more information on food allergies/addiction, refer to the reading list in Appendix B.

Be Your Own Detective: The Elimination Diet

One effective way to confirm that a specific food is causing you problems is to stop eating it for at least one week. This isn't as easy as it sounds, because if you are allergic/addicted, you may develop withdrawal symptoms as your body pleads for its usual fix of these foods. Symptoms vary from person to person and can include headache or fatigue during the first days. Back and joint aches may develop on the third day and persist for a day or two. Among the "psychological" symptoms of withdrawal are anxiety, confusion, depression, and mood swings. If you are chemically sensitive, try to avoid exposure during this week to fresh paint, new synthetic carpets, cleaning solutions, gas stoves, tobacco smoke, auto exhaust, perfumes, and shopping malls (which are filled with fumes from the formaldehyde in new clothing, furniture, and fabrics).

(A note to smokers: Do not smoke during an elimination diet. Cigarettes are loaded with chemicals that keep allergic users in a chronically reactive state. You won't be able to see the effects of the diet while you continue to smoke.)

By the end of the week, withdrawal agonies, if any, will have ceased. After that, reintroducing the suspected food(s) should produce noticeable symptoms. This is your body's way of telling you whether or not it can tolerate the food.

To test yourself, follow these directions:

1. Test only one food per meal.
2. Make a whole meal of the test food. For example, if you suspect that dairy products are the source of your problems, eat only cheese, milk, yogurt, cottage cheese; if wheat is the suspected culprit, limit yourself to hot wheat cereal, wheat toast, pancakes, or bread. Do not resume using a suspected food until after you have tested it this way. For example, don't butter your bread unless you are certain that dairy products (which include butter) are not a problem for you.
3. Take your pulse just before eating the food you are testing. Take it again five minutes after you finish and again twenty-five minutes later. A pulse twelve or more beats per minute faster or slower than what is normal for you suggests an allergic reaction to the food you are testing.
4. Make a note of any changes in the way you feel physically and emotionally. Reactions usually occur within the first hour, although some may be delayed. Be aware that if your brain chem-

istry is altered because of a reaction to the food, you may not be able to think clearly enough to accurately assess and record your reaction. I learned how difficult this can be when, after a five-day total fast (except for spring water), I tested eggs at lunch. I soon felt very sleepy and decided to take a short nap. A half hour later, I realized I was lying on the couch instead of driving back to my office. At first, I was in such a fog that I had no idea why I had dozed off at noon. As the grip of the allergic response subsided, I realized that the eggs were responsible for my reaction.

5. If possible, test the suspect foods when someone else is around. This way, if you are too muddled by an allergic reaction, your companion will be able to observe your behavior and relate it to the food you tested. I had a meeting with colleagues scheduled the day I tested wheat. After downing a stack of pancakes, I hurried off to the meeting. Driving a familiar route, I took a wrong turn, not once but twice! I was annoyed at my stupidity but never connected my mistakes to the possibility that my brain was losing its smarts in response to the wheat. When I finally arrived, I delivered my report in a halting voice, sometimes slurring my words. I was mortified by my performance. Suddenly, a close friend began to laugh. "You must be in reaction. What did you test this morning?" That embarrassing experience told me in no uncertain terms that wheat is not good for me.

6. Any uncomfortable symptoms can be partially relieved by taking two tablets of Alka-Seltzer Gold. Milk of magnesia can also help eliminate food-related problems. (Follow the directions on the label.)

7. Be sure to avoid any chemical exposure while testing a food and get plenty of fresh air. Drink only spring water, deep well water, or water that has been filtered—not tap water, which is full of chemicals. (One of our HRC clients discovered that the constant groin pain that had plagued him for years disappeared when he stopped using chlorinated water. He later found that he could turn the pain on and off by switching from spring to tap water. I have noticed that allergic people don't feel well when they drink city water treated with chlorine and other chemicals.)

Medical Testing

You can also identify food allergies through a blood test your doctor can order from Serammune Physicians' Lab in Reston, Virginia, or Immuno Nutritional Clinical Laboratories in Van Nuys, California. See Appendix C for complete addresses and telephone numbers.

The ELISA/ACT test from Serammune assesses immediate and delayed reactions to common foods and chemical compounds, pesticides, and solvents. Immuno Nutritional Laboratories offers several food-allergy panels that test from as few as 12 to as many as 125 food antigens and 24 immune complexes. Both firms also provide rotation-diet guides, books, and other educational services.

Breaking Food Allergy/Addiction

Identifying the foods that undermine your equilibrium is only half the battle. You will still find these foods appealing (in exactly the same way alcohol is appealing) because they promise a high. I doubt that your heartbeat quickens at the thought of eating green beans. But the very word "pizza" (or insert the name of your favorite food) can set something humming. That something is the anticipation of the promised high. If this seems like the effect you get from alcohol, you are beginning to understand allergy/addiction. Food addiction and alcohol or drug addiction are the same kinds of biochemical processes. This similarity explains why so many abstinent alcoholics continue to suffer physical and mental torment they expected to vanish when they stopped drinking. By kicking all of these addictions you can put an end to the physical and emotional turmoil that lures you back to one more quick fix.

Now that you understand some of the biochemical factors that underlie your need for alcohol—that overpowering buildup to drink—you can take steps to keep your brain and body in balance so you don't continually crave a chemical high to pull you out of a chronically low state.

The Total Load Concept

Imagine that you are at sea in a boat loaded with so many heavy boxes that it is sinking. You can keep afloat by tossing some boxes overboard. Your body is like that sinking boat. It has a certain threshold capacity for stress and allergen "boxes," and if you overload its capacity your physical and emotional health will suffer. Each box represents a segment of your total overload:

- One box represents food-allergy responses or high refined-sugar intake
- Another represents inhalants such as dust, mold, and pollens and chemical sensitivities to tobacco, auto exhaust, or chemicals on your job
- Another is overproliferation of *Candida albicans* yeast
- Then there is a box for all the stress in your life
- And last, but not least, is your genetic susceptibility to alcoholism

Stacked together, these boxes constitute a total environmental overload that is to blame for your physical and emotional problems. You must find a way to jettison some of them in order to get below the threshold where your physical and emotional symptoms develop.

Take the case of Bill, a recovering alcoholic who worked in a print shop. His violent temper had led to the breakup of his marriage. Now that he lived alone, Bill's diet consisted of cigarettes, colas, fast food, and coffee. Every night, while watching TV, he treated himself to a large bowl of ice cream. As the weeks and months went by, he became more depressed, more muddled in his thinking, and more and more tired. Although he was only thirty-four, Bill felt as if he were going down for the count. When he called the Health Recovery Center, he was desperate to improve the quality of his life.

We put him on a hypoglycemic diet and convinced him to give up caffeine and cut his cigarette intake in half. With biochemical repair for the damage his alcoholism had inflicted and counseling for the stress engendered by his divorce, Bill was able to reduce the environmental load on his system. To bring the load down below his personal threshold, he changed jobs so he could avoid daily exposure to the powerful chemicals in the print shop. As a result of these changes, Bill stopped craving alcohol and his violent temper disappeared. Figure 11 presents the changes Bill made to reduce the environmental load on his immune system.

Figure 11. Building-Block Theory of Immune System Breakdown from Stress Overload

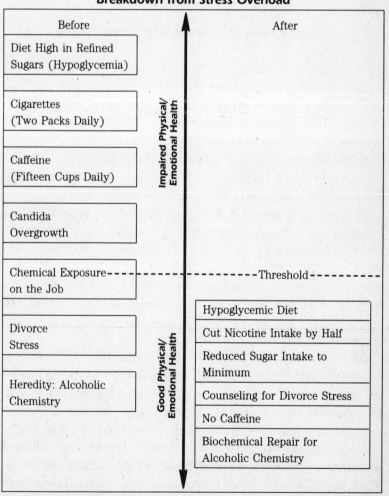

Assessing Your Personal Load

How overloaded is your immune system? You can get a pretty good idea by listing the various "boxes" you are carrying. Like Bill, you'll have to unload some in order to recover your emotional and physical equilibrium. In Appendix B you'll find a list of excellent books on food and chemical sensitivities that will give you additional information about controlling symptoms stemming from these problems.

Candida Albicans: Alcohol's Silent Partner

Bob is a typical AA member. It's Friday night, and he is attending the regular meeting at a local church. As the speaker rambles on, Bob stirs two heaping teaspoons of sugar into a large cup of coffee. He has already helped demolish a huge chocolate cake. During the two-hour meeting, Bob also drinks two cans of Coke.

As the meeting winds down, Bob finishes his second pack of cigarettes for the day. He coughs several times as he gets up to leave and resolves once again to quit smoking that weekend.

Of course, Bob doesn't quit, and by Monday his little cough has escalated into full-fledged sinusitis and bronchitis. His head aches, and he is running a temperature of 101 degrees. On Wednesday, Bob stays home from work and goes to see his family doctor, who prescribes amoxicillin, a broad-spectrum antibiotic. In a few days Bob's fever has subsided, but he still has a headache. For the next two weeks, he feels "just plain rotten." To make matters worse, the antibiotic gave him diarrhea.

Later, as he slowly recovers, Bob realizes that the infection was his third of the year; each time, it has taken longer to recover. He is worn out, worried about his health, and depressed by his physical discomfort. Bob has been depressed like this before. The only thing that seems to help is alcohol. Within days he'll fall off the wagon again.

Bob's nagging suspicion that something more than simply lowered resistance is responsible for his ill health is right on target. He has an infection with a yeast called *Candida albicans.* If you have ever been to an AA meeting, you can appreciate why candida infections are so common among both drinking and recovering alcoholics. Described by a university researcher as a "Dr. Jekyll and Mr. Hyde troublemaker" because of its elusive but destructive nature, this yeast thrives on sugar. Most alcoholics serve as tasty breeding grounds for candida because their systems are loaded with sugar.

The Nature of the Yeast

Candida albicans is a microscopic plant about the size of a red blood cell. It is a cousin to the molds that live in damp basements and is also related to the fungus that causes jock itch and athlete's foot. The textbook *Medical Mycology* describes *Candida albicans* as "mild mannered creatures incapable of producing infections in normal, healthy individuals. [A yeast] can only cause trouble in the person with weakened defenses . . . because of its rapid ability to make itself at home on mucous membranes, it can take advantage of many types of host alterations . . . The clinical manifestations of candida infections are exceedingly variable . . . [and] account for the vast majority of . . . diseases caused by yeast."

In recent years, the collection of problems related to this yeast has come to be known as candida-related complex (CRC), a term coined by allergist George Kroker, M.D. CRC embraces a variety of conditions ranging from mild to fatal. Candida can cause infections of the vagina (candida vaginitis) and mouth (thrush), as well as infections of the ears, nose, sinuses, fingers, toes, tongue, throat, esophagus, and the entire digestive tract.

Investigators at the University of Iowa report that 80 percent of the population harbors *Candida albicans*. Another researcher, David Soll, M.D., calls it a "microscopic monster" capable of inflicting infections ranging from annoying (vaginitis, jock itch) in otherwise healthy people to fatal in patients weakened by leukemia or bone-marrow transplants. Dr. Soll was the first to observe that candida is "capable of changing its looks and then changing back to its original form." This quick-change capability may allow the fungus to elude some of the body's immune-system mechanisms.

Back to Bob

Unfortunately, Bob's doctor was unaware of the problems candida can cause (this is not unusual, as I'll explain later), and the treatment he recommended actually encouraged the overgrowth. He prescribed an antibiotic that killed not only the streptococcus bacteria infecting Bob's throat and lungs, but also the normal, helpful bacteria inhabiting his digestive tract.

Once this normal balance was altered, the candida in Bob's body grew unimpeded. Candida is opportunistic; it leaps in and takes over when the body's immune defenses are down. The renegade soon covers the mucous membrane lining the small and large intestines in patches large enough to interfere with normal digestion and absorption of nutrients. The most obvious result is diarrhea, a signal that the body is trying to eliminate the candida and restore normal bacterial balance.

In Bob's case, the rapid growth of the yeast resulted in the production of toxins that altered his body's normal biochemistry and set the stage for the other disorders he developed.

Alcoholics and Candida

Results of a pilot study of the medical records of 213 patients treated at the Health Recovery Center were published in the *International Journal of Biosocial and Medical Research* in 1991. They showed that 55 percent of the women and 35 percent of the men had histories indicating probable candida overgrowth. At HRC, we use a candida questionnaire (Chart 10) developed by William Crook, M.D., to determine whether our clients are suffering from CRC. Take it to find out whether any of your symptoms could be caused by candida overgrowth.

When you talk to your doctor, explain that the yeast problem identified in the Health Recovery Center client population is systemic, not the mucocutaneous type that usually affects the vagina (yeast vaginitis) or mouth (thrush) or the invasive type that can damage the kidneys of patients on immunosuppressant drugs after organ transplants. Candida-related complex stems from many factors that involve not just yeast overgrowth but such variables as chronic stress, exces-

Chart 10. Candida Questionnaire and Score Sheet

This questionnaire is designed for adults; the scoring system isn't appropriate for children. It lists factors in your medical history that promote the growth of the common yeast, *Candida albicans* (Section A) and symptoms commonly found in individuals with yeast-connected illness (Sections B and C).

For each yes answer in Section A, circle the point score in that section. Total your score and record it in the box at the end of the section. Then move on to Sections B and C and score as directed.

Filling out and scoring this questionnaire should help you and your physician evaluate the possible role of yeasts in contributing to your health problems, but it will not provide an automatic diagnosis.

Section A: History

	Point Score
1. Have you taken tetracyclines (Sumycin, Panmycin, Vibramycin, Minocin, etc.) or other antibiotics for acne for one month (or longer)?	35
2. Have you, at any time in your life, taken other broad-spectrum antibiotics* for respiratory, urinary, or other infections (for two months or longer, or in shorter courses four or more times in a one-year period)?	35
3. Have you taken a broad-spectrum antibiotic drug*—even a single course?	6
4. Have you, at any time in your life, been bothered by persistent prostatitis, vaginitis, or other problems affecting your reproductive organs?	25
5. Have you been pregnant . . .	
Two or more times?	5
One time?	3
6. Have you taken birth-control pills . . .	
For more than two years?	15
For six months to two years?	8

*Including Keflex, ampicillin, amoxicillin, Ceclor, Bactrim, and Septra. Such antibiotics kill off the "good germs" while they're killing off those that cause infection.

Chart 10. Candida Questionnaire
and Score Sheet *(Continued)*

	Point Score
7. Have you taken prednisone, Decadron, or other cortisone-type drugs . . .	
For more than two weeks?	15
For two weeks or less?	6
8. Does exposure to perfumes, insecticides, fabric shop odors, or other chemicals provoke . . .	
Moderate to severe symptoms?	20
Mild symptoms?	5
9. Are your symptoms worse on damp, muggy days or in moldy places?	20
10. Have you had athlete's foot, ringworm, jock itch, or other chronic fungus infections of the skin or nails? Have such infections been . . .	
Severe or persistent?	20
Mild to moderate?	10
11. Do you crave sugar?	10
12. Do you crave breads?	10
13. Do you crave alcoholic beverages?	10
14. Does tobacco smoke *really* bother you?	10
Total score, Section A	

Section B: Major Symptoms

For each symptom that is present, enter the appropriate figure in the point score column:

If a symptom is occasional or mild	score 3 points
If a symptom is frequent and/or moderately severe	score 6 points
If a symptom is severe and/or disabling	score 9 points

Add the total score for this section and record it in the box at the end.

	Point Score
1. Fatigue or lethargy	
2. Feeling of being drained	
3. Poor memory	
4. Feeling spacey or unreal	
5. Inability to make decisions	
6. Numbness, burning, or tingling	
7. Insomnia	
8. Muscle aches	
9. Muscle weakness or paralysis	
10. Pain and/or swelling in joints	
11. Abdominal pain	
12. Constipation	
13. Diarrhea	
14. Bloating, belching, or intestinal gas	
15. Troublesome vaginal burning, itching, or discharge	
16. Prostatitis	
17. Impotence	
18. Loss of sexual desire or feeling	
19. Endometriosis or infertility	
20. Cramps and/or other menstrual irregularities	
21. Premenstrual tension	

Section B: Major Symptoms *(Continued)*

	Point Score
22. Attacks of anxiety or crying	
23. Cold hands or feet and/or chilliness	
24. Shaking or irritable when hungry	
Total score, Section B	

Section C: Other Symptoms†

For each symptom that is present, enter the appropriate figure in the point score column:

If a symptom is occasional or mild	score 1 point
If a symptom is frequent and/or moderately severe	score 2 points
If a symptom is severe and/or persistent	score 3 points

Add the total score for this section and record it in the box at the end.

	Point Score
1. Drowsiness	
2. Irritability or jitteriness	
3. Incoordination	
4. Inability to concentrate	
5. Frequent mood swings	
6. Headache	
7. Dizziness/loss of balance	
8. Pressure above ears, feeling of head swelling	
9. Tendency to bruise easily	
10. Chronic rashes or itching	
11. Psoriasis or recurrent hives	
12. Indigestion or heartburn	
13. Food sensitivity or intolerance	

†While the symptoms in this section occur commonly in patients with yeast-connected illness, they also occur commonly in patients who do not have candida.

	Point Score
14. Mucus in stools	
15. Rectal itching	
16. Dry mouth or throat	
17. Rash or blisters in mouth	
18. Bad breath	
19. Foot, hair, or body odor not relieved by washing	
20. Nasal congestion or postnasal drip	
21. Nasal itching	
22. Sore throat	
23. Laryngitis, loss of voice	
24. Cough or recurrent bronchitis	
25. Pain or tightness in chest	
26. Wheezing or shortness of breath	
27. Urinary frequency, urgency, or incontinence	
28. Burning on urination	
29. Spots in front of eyes or erratic vision	
30. Burning or tearing of eyes	
31. Recurrent infections or fluid in ears	
32. Ear pain or deafness	
Total score, Section C	
Total score, Section B	
Total score, Section A	
Grand total score	

Section C: Other Symptoms *(Continued)*

The grand total score will help you and your physician decide if your health problems are yeast-connected. Scores in women will run higher as seven items in the questionnaire apply exclusively to women, while only two apply exclusively to men.

Yeast-connected health problems are almost certainly present in women with scores over 180 and in men with scores over 140.

Yeast-connected health problems are probably present in women with scores over 120 and in men with scores over 90.

Yeast-connected health problems are possibly present in women with scores over 60 and in men with scores over 40.

With scores of less than 60 in women and 40 in men, yeasts are less likely to be the cause of health problems.

---

sive sugar intake, the use of broad-spectrum antibiotics, lowered immunity, environmental pollution, and, in some patients, prolonged use of oral contraceptives and corticosteroids.

Treating Candida

At Health Recovery Center we treat CRC with nystatin powder, a drug that requires a physician's prescription. The physician on our staff usually prescribes one-quarter teaspoon dissolved in one-half glass of water to be taken before each meal and at bedtime for at least two months (sometimes for as long as four months). Clients with CRC who also have sinusitis or nose and ear infections will also need to take the prescription antifungal drug diflucan for three weeks.

Bob scored high on his candida questionnaire and a laboratory candida antibody assay. After six weeks of treatment for CRC, his depression had vanished, his energy was on the upswing, and his cravings for alcohol and sugar had disappeared. "I haven't felt this good for ten years," he exulted. "Even my postnasal drip is gone."

Bob did recover, but he had to change many of his ways. Today, when he attends AA meetings, he drinks herbal tea. He stopped smoking and brings his own snacks to meetings—whole grain bread with almond butter, a few pistachios and filberts, carrots and celery sticks. Putting sugar out of his life eliminated the cravings that had kept him on the edge of relapse for years.

Be Prepared for Resistance

Don't be surprised if your doctor is not impressed with Bob's story, the results of your CRC questionnaire, and your determination to have yourself tested for CRC. Many physicians still adhere to the old (and incorrect) view that *Candida albicans* accounts only for disorders in the intestinal tract, not for disorders that occur elsewhere in the body. If your doctor dismisses the notion that CRC may be to blame for otherwise unexplained symptoms, refer him to the candida-related complex readings in Appendix B.

Eventually, I'm sure that skeptical physicians will begin to recognize and treat the physical and mental havoc CRC can create. But you can't wait for medical thinking to evolve. You need help now. To find a sympathetic physician, telephone the International Health Foundation at (800) 372-7665 or the American Academy of Environmental Medicine at (303) 622-9755.

We have now covered all of the biochemical, nutritional, and allergy-related problems that can underlie alcoholism and complicate recovery. Your repair program is complete. You are no longer drinking, and you no longer crave alcohol. You are eating a new, healthy diet designed to correct any problems you had with hypoglycemia. You have restored the vital nutrients alcohol had depleted, and your body and brain are again functioning normally. And now you have identified chemical sensitivities and/or food allergies that so often accompany alcoholism. If necessary, you are en route to recovery from CRC.

What next?

Now you must ensure that your recovery is permanent. The following chapter contains the HRC aftercare plan, the strategy you will rely on in the years to come to solidify the gains you have made in the past six weeks. You will also learn how to stop smoking with the aid of nutrients that can diminish and even dispell your craving for nicotine.

You should feel proud and happy to have reached this point in your recovery program. Now it is time to think seriously of the future. You are ready to bid a permanent farewell to alcoholism and take charge of the rest of your life.

Twelve

Week Seven: Planning the Future

Not long ago I had lunch with a former client, a successful young builder. Jim was brimming with health and energy. He told me that his business was doing so well that he could take time off to race cars at tracks around the country. Listening to him, it was hard to believe that just four short years ago Jim's life was at a standstill, bogged down by lack of motivation and mental confusion.

Jim had completed another treatment program before coming to Health Recovery Center, but no one there had told him he couldn't live on ice cream, coffee, and cigarettes. The intervening years had been miserable for him. He had resumed drinking. The more sugar and alcohol he used, the worse his cravings became. He was also subject to dramatic mood swings, complained of fatigue, and said he often felt too spacey to function. His intelligence and talent were obvious, but they were going to waste as he continued to drink.

Now the picture is quite different. Jim has been through some rough times since I first met him, including a painful divorce, but he has managed to weather it admirably. I asked him what has kept him sober over the years.

"I never knew I could feel this good," he replied. "Now that I do, I would be a fool to deliberately destroy myself by letting alcoholism take over again." Even today, Jim continues to use the recovery strategy he learned at HRC. It has served him well. It can do the same for you.

If you have been making the changes I have recommended in this book, undoubtedly you too have begun to feel healthy and energetic. To prove to yourself how far you have come in six short weeks, I would like you to retest yourself for any current symptoms by again completing Health Recovery Center's symptometer (Chart 11). Compare your new score with your score from Week One (Chart 3). The results will confirm the improvement in your health. You may still have a few lingering symptoms, but they will disappear gradually over the next few weeks or months as you follow your aftercare plan. In this chapter, I'll give you the strategies you'll need to maintain your sobriety and further improve your general health. And, at last, I'll give you HRC's tested and effective plan for overcoming one last addiction—your dependency on nicotine. If you're still smoking, the time has come to quit!

Do you remember the relapse studies I cited in Chapter 1—the ones demonstrating that more than 75 percent of alcoholics resume drinking only a year after treatment? Those formidable odds can defeat the incentive to depend on sheer willpower. But you have at your command powerful recovery tools that will enable you to beat those odds and continue on the path to renewed energy and health.

In the pages ahead you will find a plan to follow during this first crucial year. Like your repair program, you will need to personalize this regime to suit your individual needs. It encompasses physical, psychological, and personal-growth strategies you can use to maintain and build on the gains you have made in the past six weeks.

Chart 11. The HRC Symptometer
Week Seven

	Frequency			
Symptom	**Never 0**	**Mild 1**	**Moderate 2**	**Severe 3**
1. Cravings for alcohol	——	——	——	——
2. Uses alcohol regularly	——	——	——	——
3. Tendency to allergies, asthma, hay fever, rashes	——	——	——	——
4. Bad dreams	——	——	——	——
5. No dream recall	——	——	——	——
6. Unstable moods, frequent mood swings	——	——	——	——
7. Blurred vision	——	——	——	——
8. Frequent thirst	——	——	——	——
9. Bruises easily	——	——	——	——
10. Confusion	——	——	——	——
11. Nervous stomach	——	——	——	——
12. Poor sleep, insomnia, waking up during the night	——	——	——	——
13. Nervous exhaustion	——	——	——	——
14. Indecision	——	——	——	——
15. Can't work under pressure	——	——	——	——
16. Cravings for sweets	——	——	——	——
17. Depression	——	——	——	——
18. Feelings of suspicion, paranoia	——	——	——	——
19. Light-headedness, dizziness	——	——	——	——
20. Anxiety	——	——	——	——

Chart 11. The HRC Symptometer
Week Seven (*Continued*)

Symptom	Never 0	Mild 1	Moderate 2	Severe 3
21. Fearfulness	___	___	___	___
22. Tremors, shakes	___	___	___	___
23. Night sweats	___	___	___	___
24. Heart palpitations	___	___	___	___
25. Compulsive, obsessive, driven	___	___	___	___
26. Manic-depressive (cyclical mood changes)	___	___	___	___
27. Suicidal thoughts	___	___	___	___
28. Irritability, sudden anger	___	___	___	___
29. Lack of energy	___	___	___	___
30. Magnifies insignificant events	___	___	___	___
31. Poor memory	___	___	___	___
32. Inability to concentrate	___	___	___	___
33. Sleepy after meals or late in the afternoon	___	___	___	___
34. Chronic worrier	___	___	___	___
35. Difficulty awakening in the morning	___	___	___	___
Column Totals	___	___	___	___
Test Total	___	___	___	___

INSTRUCTIONS: Check off each symptom in one of the columns to indicate the degree of severity that applies to you. Zero means never, one means mild, two means moderate, and three means severe. Add up the number of checks in each column and multiply by the number printed at the top of each column. Total score equals the sum of all columns. (Scores over 35 are significant.)

Physical Strategies That Heal

Your most important task during the coming months is to avoid all drugs (except those prescribed by your doctor). That most definitely includes alcohol. You must also continue to stay away from nicotine, caffeine, and over-the-counter drugs that contain alcohol (read the labels carefully). Now that your system has been cleansed of substances that sapped your health and energy, your goal is to keep it that way. The alternative is an internal toxic environment that makes you need a lift. By now you understand that the quick fix provided by ice cream, caffeine, or cigarettes can lead to the ultimate best fix: alcohol.

I also want to remind that the one-quarter of HRC clients who relapse after completing treatment have one thing in common: *they continued to smoke cigarettes.* Our findings duplicate a 1978 study published in the *Journal of Addictive Behavior* that correlated smoking with relapse rates. Please believe me when I tell you that you must treat all of your drug dependencies simultaneously if you hope to free yourself permanently from the powerful vise of physical addiction. Years of experience has taught me that leaving just one drug in place can undo all the gains made by following the HRC treatment plan.

There is no more deadly drug than nicotine. It kills more Americans than alcohol and all other drugs combined. Today, about 25 percent of all Americans smoke, but 83 percent of all alcoholics are smokers. The abstinent drinkers who can't manage to quit smoking are in danger of returning to alcohol. I don't want you to get caught in this trap, so let's take a look at how you're going to stop smoking once and for all.

Kicking the Cigarette Habit

Giving up cigarettes and nicotine can be done. Millions of ex-smokers have confronted this moment and forged ahead successfully. They were no stronger than you are now, and you have the advantage of a strategy that works. I've seen it succeed again and again. If you let it it will work for you. You can't afford not to.

Set a target date to quit smoking—two weeks from today. As the date approaches, take the following steps:

1. Continue to avoid caffeine, junk food, and refined sugars.
2. Stick to your daily exercise program. It will help you counteract weight gain when you stop smoking.
3. Cut down on cigarettes over the two-week period before your quit date. This will be easier if you take sodium/potassium bicarbonate (Alka-Seltzer Gold) to alkalize your system and reduce your craving for nicotine. You can take two tablets every four hours but no more than eight tablets in any twenty-four-hour period.
4. Avoid red meats, organ meats, cranberries, plums, and prunes (they promote the acidity you are trying to neutralize with Alka-Seltzer Gold).
5. Drink at least six glasses of water a day.

Some of the nutrients you are taking will help you rid your system of nicotine and reduce your cravings. In some cases, you may have to increase your dosage slightly. Read through the following descriptions to see how the nutrients listed can help you and to determine how much you should be taking.

- GABA (gamma-aminobutyric acid): As you now know, GABA has a calming and centering effect. Smokers accustomed to nicotine's stress-reducing properties (it lowers reactions to outside stimuli by altering certain neurotransmitters in the brain) find that GABA helps deliver the same results. An adequate source of GABA is the Calm Kids formula recommended on page 181. If you are already taking Calm Kids, do not duplicate the dosage. If not, take six capsules per day, two with each meal.
- Glutamine: Did you know that cigarettes are up to 75 percent sugar? Tobacco is cured with beet, corn, and cane sugars. As long as these sugars are entering their bloodstreams with any regularity, hypoglycemic smokers won't be able to bring their blood sugar under control. Glutamine, an alternative source of glucose, can alleviate hypoglycemic reactions among smokers. You are already

taking enough glutamine in your adjusted nutrient plan. Do not duplicate.

- Zinc: Smokers are usually deficient in zinc because the body uses a lot of it to remove the buildup of cadmium, a metal contained in cigarette papers (it makes them white). Increase your total zinc intake to fifty milligrams per day for six weeks.

- B complex: These vitamins can help allay the nervousness that develops as nicotine leaves the system. Cigarettes seriously deplete vitamin B_1 (thiamine).

In addition to these nutrients, you can quench nicotine cravings with Nicorette gum, available with a doctor's prescription. Results of a study published April 1987 in the *Journal of the American Medical Association* showed that Nicorette doubles the success rate among smokers trying to quit. The gum provides a minimum dose of nicotine that alleviates the irritability and anxiety that often occur during withdrawal. The study also found that weight gain is minimal when Nicorette is used by smokers trying to quit.

Nicoril capsules, which contain lobelia and other herbs, can also help reduce your craving for nicotine. The manufacturer offers a full refund if Nicoril does not help you break your cigarette habit. If your local health store does not carry Nicoril, contact Phyto-Pharmacia, P.O. Box 1348, Green Bay, WI 54305. Follow the directions on the package when taking Nicoril.

Your Diet During Recovery

Eliminating refined sugars, including alcohol, from your diet has banished your hypoglycemic symptoms. To keep them at bay, your love affair with sugar must never be rekindled. If you succumb to the temptation of these "treats," sugar addiction will sneak back into your life, bringing with it the old fatigue and mood swings. If you avoid refined sugars for a few years, your blood sugar should return to normal and stay there. I think of the tendency toward sugar addiction as a sleeping giant. An occasional treat won't awaken it. But you must guard against zooming past occasional right back to daily. As a recovering hypoglycemic myself, I have found that I can (and do!) have an ice cream cone once a year while on vacation. I also give myself a little leeway at Christmas, but certain rules remain ironclad. I *never* eat chocolates or other kinds of candies, and I still only buy baked goods sweetened with fruit juice instead of refined sugars. (You can find these goodies at food co-ops and in supermarket health sections.)

Less easy to cope with are the sugars in fruit salads, baked beans, and other foods you may be served by friends or find on restaurant menus. You need a strategy to politely decline or avoid these dishes. Think about your choices in advance before you open a restaurant menu. With friends, a polite but firm no thank you should do the trick. It's certainly easier than giving in and having to break your sugar addiction all over again.

You can maintain the gains you've made during your recovery program by following the hypoglycemic diet for alcoholics at the end of this chapter. It includes all forms of whole wheat and dairy products. II ADH/THIQ and omega-6 EFA deficient alcohol biotypes should have no problems with foods containing either wheat or dairy products, but allergic/addicted biotypes must continue to avoid any foods to which they are sensitive. (You can retest these foods in six months using the instructions in Chapter 11. By then, you may be able to handle them normally. Even so, try not to eat these foods every day. Instead, limit your consumption to once every four days in order to avoid a recurrence of your addictive response.)

HRC's Hypoglycemic Diet for Alcoholics

Suggested Daily Menus

Breakfast:

Two eggs or yogurt

One slice protein bread or ¼ cup oatmeal, millet, buckwheat, or whole-wheat cereal

One glass of milk or other acceptable beverage

or

One pat butter
One slice natural cheese

or

Fresh fruit in season
Handful of raw nuts: almonds, sesame seeds, or pumpkin seeds
One cup of yogurt

or

One cup cooked cereal: millet, buckwheat, whole wheat, or oats
One pat of sweet butter

Midmorning Snack:
Five to ten raw almonds or other raw, unroasted nuts

or

One piece fresh fruit: pear, pineapple, papaya, melon, or a bowl of
    cherries
One slice cheddar or other natural cheese

or

½ large or 1 small avocado

or

Tomato or V-8 juice 8 to 12 oz.

or

Orange juice or grapefruit juice (diluted 2:1 with spring water)

Lunch:
One slice whole-grain bread
One pat butter
One slice natural cheese

or

Beans and brown rice with fresh tomato, onion, garlic

or

½ cup drained, canned salmon, tuna, or sardines
Small vegetable salad

or

Any breakfast choice

or

Hamburger patty with melted cheese
Tossed salad with natural dressing or avocado
Sautéed mushrooms with butter
Beverage
Fresh peach

or

Bowl of freshly prepared vegetable, mushroom, pea, or lentil soup

or

Any other cooked or steamed vegetable dish such as green beans,
carrots, broccoli, cauliflower, zucchini

Midafternoon Snack:
Same as midmorning snack

Dinner:
Broiled chicken (remove skin)
½ baked potato
Green or wax beans
One slice whole-grain bread (with one to two pats butter)
Mixed raw vegetables
Strawberries
Herbal tea

After-Dinner Snack:
Same as midmorning snack

Foods to Avoid

Beverages

Alcoholic beverages

Caffeinated Beverages:

  Cocoa

  Coffee

  Cola

Decaffeinated beverages

Diet soft drinks

Ovaltine

Soft drinks

Strong tea

Desserts

Cake

Chocolate

Cookies

Custard

Dessert topping

Ice cream

Jell-O

Pastry

Pie

Puddings

Fruit

Dried fruits (raisins, dates, etc.)

Fruits canned in syrup

Grains

"Enriched" white flours:

  Breads

  Cereal (dry)

Crackers (white)

Grits

Pancakes (from white)

Pizza

Pretzels

Rolls

Waffles

(Avoid enriched white flours in any form. Use whole-grain flours.)

Meats

Canned meats

Cold cuts

Hot dogs

Salami

Sausages

Bacon

(These are usually packed with some form of sugar as a preservative. Check labels for exceptions.)

Pasta

Macaroni

Noodles

Spaghetti

(Unless made with whole grains)

Sweets

Artificial sweeteners

Candy

Caramel

Chewing gum

Honey

Jam

Jelly

Malt

Marmalade

Molasses

Sugar

Syrup

Other forms of sugar: dextrose, fructose, glucose, hexitol, lactose, maltose mannitol, sorbitol, sucrose

Vegetables

Potato chips or fries

Rice (white)

Pickes (sweet)

Relishes (sweet)

Allowable Foods

Beverages

Apricot juice

Carrot juice

Clear broth

Grapefruit juice

Herb teas

Lemon juice

Lime juice

Loganberry juice

Milk

Orange juice

Pineapple juice

Raspberry juice

Sauerkraut juice

Tangerine juice

Tomato juice

V-8 juice

Vegetable juice

Dilute all fruit juices 2:1
  with spring water

Cheeses

Cream cheese and cottage cheese have roughly one-half the protein value of most other cheeses. Do not use processed cheese, cheese spreads, or squeeze-bottle cheese. Cheese does have a high fat and sodium content.

Fats

Fats are essential for steroid production, and the fats in butter, cream, milk (if tolerated), and salad oil contribute to a well-balanced diet, as do fats present in other natural foods.

Fruit (fresh)

Apples
Apricots
Avocado
Blueberries
Cantaloupe
Casaba melon
Cherries
Coconut (fresh)
Fruit salad (without grapes)
Grapefruit
Grapes (eat sparingly,
    high in fructose)

Honeydew melon
Lemon
Lime
Muskmelon
Oranges
Peaches
Pears
Pineapple
Plums
Raspberries
Rhubarb (no sugar added)
Strawberries
Tangerines

Although bananas contain 23 percent fructose carbohydrates, one banana a day is permitted because of its high potassium content.

Nuts and Seeds

Almonds
Brazil nuts
Peanuts
Pecans
Pumpkin seeds
Sesame seeds
Sunflower seeds
Walnuts

These are good sources of protein. Use raw nuts and seeds only. The roasting process changes the fat content of nuts and seeds to form free radicals, which are potential carcinogens, so avoid roasted products.

Protein

Chicken and other fowl
Eggs
Fish
Meat

Shellfish
Tofu (soy)

Salt

Allowed in moderate amounts. Consider Morton's Lite Salt, which is half potassium, half sodium and will cut your sodium intake by 50 percent.

Sprouts

Alfalfa
Bean

Vegetables (fresh)

Artichokes (globe or French)
Asparagus
Beans (green or wax)
Beets
Broccoli
Cabbage
Cauliflower
Celery
Cucumbers
Lettuce
Mushrooms
Olives
Onions (green or raw)
Parsley
Peppers
Pickles (dill or sour)
Pimentos
Peas (green or edible pod)
Potatoes
Radishes
Rutabaga
Sauerkraut
Soybeans
Spinach
Squash (Hubbard or winter)
Tomatoes
Water chestnuts
Zucchini

Whole grains

Barley
Buckwheat
Millet
Oatmeal
Rice (brown or wild)
Whole wheat

The Rewards of Exercise

Your exercise program can boost your self-esteem and enhance your energy. Alcoholic or not, regular exercise offers many rewards:

- You will find it easier to cope with stress
- You will look more radiant, move more gracefully, stand taller, and look more youthful
- You will burn calories faster and look trimmer
- You will eat less and find junk foods less appealing
- You will relieve tension and banish mild down moods
- Your body and mind will function better: the aging process will slow as your heart and lung function, digestion, and elimination improve, and your immune system will become stronger, and your joints, more flexible

Designing Your Exercise Program

The best exercise plan is one you can stick to. It does not have to be strenuous. One-half hour of brisk walking, biking, or swimming at least four times a week is all you need. However, if you have any athletic inclination, you may find that you want more exercise.

The usual excuse for not exercising is lack of time. Well, exercising need not take time out of your day. I work out at home on my trampoline or exercise bike while I watch television. I prefer not leaving home to exercise, but many people need the motivation a group provides. So design your own plan, join a gym, or enroll in an aerobics class. But whatever you do, make sure it is convenient, so that you'll participate on a regular basis.

Most recovering alcoholics find that they have a lot of time on their hands, time they used to spend drinking. An exercise program can fit right in.

Your Maintenance Nutrient Program

During the last week of the HRC program, clients begin to ask how long they have to take all those vitamins. Or they complain that they can't afford to keep replacing their nutrients. Or they tell me that they love the way one particular nutrient makes them feel but that they no longer need all the rest.

At this point, they are feeling great. As the program ends, some of our clients think they can walk on water and that their continued sobriety is assured. True, many biochemical improvements are underway, but the change is not yet complete. It is an evolving process that, over time, will yield a very high level of health. But at this point I must caution you that your new life-style is still tenuous. You have not yet finished building the strong habits that guarantee long-term success. It would be foolish to abandon your nutrient program now. You need a scaled-down maintenance plan to carry you through the next months. The maintenance doses given in Chart 12 apply to all alcohol biotypes.

Your HRC aftercare plan should also include any of the specific repair formulas you have been using. Continue to take them at the doses recommended for three more months. Then discontinue for three weeks to see how you feel. If any symptoms return, resume taking the formula for another three months and then stop again to determine whether you need further treatment.

Use Chart 12 to add these formulas to your maintenance list. Remember to add up the amounts of each nutrient you take. Consult the tables in Chapter 9 to determine the safe maximum amount of all vitamins and minerals. Do not exceed the therapeutic dose recommended.

Aftercare Reminders

If you are taking a prescription drug for high blood pressure or candida-related complex or have been given desensitizing drops by your clinical ecologist, be sure to keep your next doctor's appointment. Following through when no one is monitoring you is often difficult in the early stages of recovery. DO IT!

Chart 12. Six-Month Nutrient Maintenance Plan (All Biotypes)

Combination Total	Nutrient	Number of Capsules	Daily Dose
	Glutamine—to stop cravings for alcohol/sugar; continue to use as needed to control cravings (500 mg)	2 capsules midmorning and 2 capsules midafternoon (between meals)	2,000 mg
	Free-form amino acids—to rebuild neurotransmitters (750 mg)	1 capsule three times a day between meals	2,250 mg
	Vitamin C—for the immune system (1,000 mg)	1 capsule with each meal	3,000 mg
	Multi-vitamin/mineral formula	2 capsules at breakfast 2 capsules at dinner	
	Vitamin A (palmitate)		16,000 IU
	Vitamin B_1 (thiamine)		80 mg
	Vitamin B_2 (riboflavin)		40 mg
	Vitamin B_3 (niacinamide)		120 mg
	Vitamin B_5 (pantothenic acid)		400 mg

Chart 12. Six-Month Nutrient
Maintenance Plan (All Biotypes) *(Continued)*

Combination Total	Nutrient	Number of Capsules	Daily Dose
	Vitamin B_6 (pyridoxine)		120 mg
	Pyridoxal-5′-phosphate		4 mg
	Vitamin B_{12} (cobalamine)		320 mcg
	Tryptophan		120 mg
	Folic acid		240 mcg
	Biotin		320 mcg
	PABA		160 mg
	Vitamin E		320 IU
	Calcium		200 mg
	Magnesium		200 mg
	Potassium		80 mg
	Mangenese		12 mg
	Zinc		24 mg
	Copper		1.2 mg
	Selenium		160 mcg
	Vanadium		160 mcg
	Molybdenum		160 mcg
	Glutamic acid		160 mcg
	Chromium		320 mcg
	Iron		16 mg

Chart 12. Six-Month Nutrient
Maintenance Plan (All Biotypes) *(Continued)*

Combination Total	Nutrient	Number of Capsules	Daily Dose
	Fortified flax omega-3 EFA continue unless eating fish 4 × weekly	1 heap tblsp daily	
	Efamol—lifts depression in EFA deficient alcoholics. This biotype must continue Efamol use indefinitely; others continue for six months (500 mg)	2 capsules with each meal	3,000 mg
	Antioxidant complex— needed by those with chemical sensitivities; builds up weak immune systems	1 capsule daily with food	
36,000 IU	Vitamin A (beta-carotene)		20,000 IU
	Glutathione		60 mg
	Methionine		40 mg
470 IU	Vitamin E		150 IU
	Dimethylglycine		80 mg
	Cysteine		80 mg
3,040 mg	Vitamin C		40 mg
34 mg	Zinc		10 mg

Chart 12. Six-Month Nutrient
Maintenance Plan (All Biotypes) *(Continued)*

Combination Total	Nutrient	Number of Capsules	Daily Dose
190 mcg	Selenium		30 mcg
	Ubiquinone		500 mcg
	Lipoic acid		2.5 mg
1,120–2,120 mg	Tryptophan*— for sleep, if available (500 mg)	2–4 capsules at bedtime	1,000–2,000 mg
	or		
	GABA Plus—for sleep (500 mg)	1–3 capsules at bedtime	500–1,500 mg
	Pancreatic enzymes—to aid digestion and absorption of foods; needed by allergic/addicted biotypes and those with candida-related complex (425 mg)	1–2 capsules with each meal	1,275–2,550 mg

*Use only if the FDA lifts the current ban on its sale.

Additional Nutrient Formulas

Combination Total	Nutrient	Number of Capsules	Daily Dose

Psychological Strategies That Work

Until now, the tools suggested in this chapter have been designed to help you avoid primary physical cravings for alcohol. But there are secondary, psychological triggers that can and will sabotage you if you let them. These secondary triggers arise from outside, not inside, the body. A few examples:

- Spending time with drinking buddies
- Sudden stress (such as a fight with your spouse)
- Financial setbacks
- Permission-giving self-talk: "I feel so good I think I could handle a few drinks now"
- Parties or social gatherings where alcohol is served
- Intense negative emotions such as self-pity, anger, or fear

To help you avoid these emotional pitfalls, I am going to provide you with the most powerful weapons I have discovered during my sixteen years in this field.

Build Yourself a Support System

You are not the first alcoholic to wrestle with the temptation to drink again. Others have won the battle with successful strategies you can and should adopt to help you through the years ahead. Friends who understand your needs and your pain can be an enormous help. You can also find the support you need through Alcoholics Anonymous or Women for Sobriety, both of which have groups in most communities. I cannot overemphasize the importance of these invaluable human resources. Nowhere else can you find others who have a gut-level understanding and appreciation of what you have been through. They are waiting for your call. Make it today.

Consider Therapy

Throughout this book I have explained repeatedly what therapy cannot do for recovering alcoholics. Therapy *cannot* repair your alcohol-altered brain and nervous system or banish the depression, unstable moods, and cravings that stem from the biochemical changes alcohol brings about. But therapy *can* help you with a number of painful problems. Such serious emotional issues as childhood incest or physical/emotional abuse by your mate demand attention. Without help, emotional problems can drive you to drink again to cover up the pain. Don't risk relapse by neglecting emotion-charged issues.

Your first step in this direction will be to find the right therapist. This is not as simple as it sounds. I believe you will benefit most rapidly by working with someone who uses rational-emotive (cognitive) therapy. This approach focuses on current choices rather than past failures. Within this psychological framework, you'll learn how to deal effectively with your anger, self-hate, fear, worry, emotional stress, and assertiveness.

If you have financial problems, don't assume that you can't afford therapy. In most areas, United Way organizations (such as Family and Children's Services) can arrange for treatment on a sliding reimbursement scale based on your ability to pay.

Create a Circle of Sober Friends

The cruelest advice counselors must dispense concerns some of the most important people in your life, your drinking buddies. Often, they are your only friends, and you find yourself in a no-win situation: if you socialize with drinkers, eventually you will drink. On the other hand, life without friends is lonely and can bring on self-pity that can drive you to drink. The solution is to seek out social activities with any and all sober acquaintances and relatives who appeal to you. Look for them at work, in your neighborhood, church circle, classes. As you contemplate new friendships, your self-talk may be negative: "Not at my age" or "Who wants my company?" Remember that each of us suffers from some degree of self-hatred. We all tell ourselves, "I'm not good enough." The reality is that most people will welcome your friendship. If you doubt that, consider your own receptivity to new acquaintances. Few of us willingly pass up the opportunity to make a new friend. To protect your sobriety, it is essential that you find and cultivate people you like who live a sober life and know how to enjoy themselves.

Involving Loved Ones in Recovery

If you have a mate who will accompany you on your journey to recovery, you are fortunate indeed. Cooperation at home can make all the difference between successful and unsuccessful recovery. Rifts and hurt feelings can persist unless your mate comes to understand alcoholism as a disease that alters brain chemistry and causes unacceptable but not intentional behavior. In a traditional treatment approach, the families of patients gather to voice their pain and heap their resentment on the alcoholic. Can you imagine relatives of patients with diabetes or cancer meeting that way? It would be regarded as inhumane, unthinkable. Families need to understand the true nature of alcohol addiction so that time together can be used for healing, not accusations. See Appendix B for a list of books that can help you all make progress in this direction.

Ideally, your spouse and children will choose to share your basic diet. Giving up junk foods, additives, and refined sugars will be good for the whole family. Sharing your B-complex vitamins will provide your overstressed mate with the same calming effect you now enjoy.

Codependency: Fact or Fiction?

The codependency concept holds that mates of alcoholics are equally to blame for their spouses' "alcoholic" behavior and are guilty of "enabling" their drinking by covering up to children, employers, bankers, creditors. In light of what we now know about the genetic basis of alcoholism and the physical toll it takes on its victims, feeling responsible for your mate's alcoholism becomes absurd. Anyone who has lived with an alcoholic soon comes to understand how powerless he or she is to stop alcoholic behavior. A spouse need not take on the additional burden of guilt for a mate's illness. Women especially have been all too willing to accept a share of the "blame" for alcoholism. To such "codependents," I suggest that it is not difficult to see who the sick member of the family is. The mate brings strength, not weakness, to the relationship. Adding this strength to the recovery strategies presented in this book vastly enhances the alcoholic's prospects for regaining sobriety and physical and emotional health.

Personal-Growth Strategies That Work

People who stop drinking have a lot of time on their hands. Some react with boredom and listlessness. NOT YOU! Being wiser, you'll look upon this precious commodity as a gift and use it to invest in your future happiness. On the medallion we present to each HRC graduate (Figure 12) is the motto "Total Recovery: Mind, Body, Spirit." Each side of the triangle represents an essential aspect of our humanity. To neglect any of the three can jeopardize your recovery.

"I Don't Need Religion, Thank You"

That is what I hear from many HRC clients when I inquire about spiritual needs. I tell them that spirituality is not necessarily religious belief. It is an awareness of a center within that sustains us and gives us the strength to conquer our insecurities. AA members describe this spirituality as "God as you have come to know Him." To some, this may be limited to communing with nature in a woodsy setting; to others, it is an awareness of an inner core—"God," if you will—that defines us and, despite our frailties, enables us to perceive our true natures. It is no accident that most HRC clients who proclaim at the outset that they have no spirituality find that by Week Six they have stirred the ashes of their deeper selves. My personal belief is that the physical and emotional damage alcoholism causes pulls down all sorts of wires in the mind, making communication with our higher selves impossible. With healing, the wires are repaired and the signals again transmit.

It would be foolhardy for me to give you more than general directions toward spiritual nourishment. In this respect, each of us follows an individual path. But I can pass along strategies for building spiritual health that HRC clients have chosen for themselves:

- Setting aside time for daily meditation
- Reading inspirational books

Figure 12. HRC Medallion

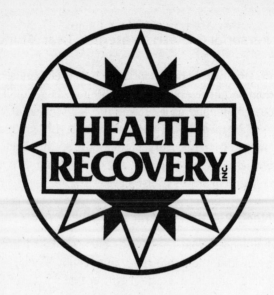

- Seeking a friendly faith community
- Attending religious services
- Taking time off for a retreat in a peaceful setting
- Forgiving others, sharing love with others

Often Health Recovery Center clients tell us that previous counselors have advised them to cut themselves off from parents who mistreated them as children. Although that may be possible physically, it is nearly impossible to sever spiritual and emotional bonds with parents. If one or both of your parents was actively alcoholic when you were growing up, you may have a lot of painful memories. Not many illnesses destroy sanity as dramatically as alcoholism. Now that you understand the effects of this disease, you can see your parent's behavior in light of the unstable brain chemistry alcoholism promotes.

At Health Recovery Center, we encourage clients to renew relationships with parents whenever possible in order to knock down walls built over the years. Sharing your love with others is a precious spiritual experience. Don't be afraid to tell those dear to you that you love them.

What Are You Going to Be When You Grow Up?

Your personal-growth strategies should include your secret ambitions for yourself. It is never to late to follow your dreams. But to make them come true, you must set your goals and devise a plan of action.

The failures caused by your illness are behind you now. Unfortunately, you are still programmed to think of yourself in the old way. Your new self-image will come with practice. A classic book that can teach you how to change your view of yourself is *Psycho-Cybernetics* by Maxwell Maltz, Ph.D. Another excellent book that can help you find self-love and self-esteem is Louise Hay's *You Can Heal Your Life*. Restructuring your life externally by pursuing more education or career changes will succeed only if you rebuild your internal capacity for living. At this point, you should be ready to take on this important task to enhance and preserve your recovery.

As you grow, you will probably have lots of new ideas about your career possibilities. Most universities have career testing programs that can help you pinpoint your strengths. If you have the aptitude and want a new career, now is the time to go for it!

Education: Your Ticket to the Future

There has never been a better time in history to learn something special and be someone special. You can enroll in business school or vocational-technical courses, take college courses on weekends or in the evenings, even apply for college credits for life experience. In time, you can attain your goals and reshape your life. After all, the years will go by whether or not you choose to move forward. I have watched certain clients learn that lesson and apply it to their own lives. Many who start with the most serious handicaps have ultimately made the greatest strides. I particularly remember Gerrie, the black sheep of her family. Her brothers and sisters were all overachievers who held prestigious jobs while Gerrie bounced from one alcoholism treatment program to another. The Health Recovery Center program was her seventh attempt at recovery. Her family had seen her fail so many times that no one volunteered to participate with her as a concerned other. But Gerrie turned out to be a real survivor. She wholeheartedly plunged into the program and surprised her entire family with her success. Now, four years later, she remains alcohol free. Her daughter recently telephoned to thank me for the "miracle" that freed Gerrie from alcoholism. Gerrie is about to graduate from college with a degree in nursing. She had propelled herself from the welfare rolls to a whole new life because she never lost sight of her dreams and never doubted her ability to make them come true.

The limits we place on ourselves are self-invented. We can do as much as we decide to do. So get started:

- Call your school for a brochure
- Explore financial-aid possibilities (grants and student loans)
- Make an appointment to talk to a vocational counselor
- Start now, even if you can only take one class per semester.

And What About Love?

Alcoholism counselors often discourage their clients from getting in-volved in intimate relationships immediately after treatment. They have in mind the kind of conquest relationships where self-gratifica-tion is the main object of the game or where one partner endows the other with a projected image of what this loved one "should" be. In both cases, the inevitable outcome is disappointment and the kind of emotional letdown that can send you back to numbing your misery with alcohol.

They are correct to urge caution. Go very slowly. Real love usually comes when you least expect it and when you are able to attract the right person for you. You will know when this happens. Real love makes us happy, not jealous, sad, or feeling that we don't measure up. Beware of relationships that you find painful or unhappy. As a test of whether a relationship is healthy, ask yourself the following questions:

- Are you continually preoccupied with the person you "love," trying to please him/her at your own expense?
- Do you depend on your mate for good feelings? Do your moods alter according to your mate's moods? Has your sense of self-worth diminished?
- Does most of your life revolve around trying to please your mate? Are you afraid that making waves will cost you the relationship?
- Do you feel an obsessive need to possess your mate's affections in order to define yourself as a worthwhile human being?

If you answer yes to any of these questions, the relationship is not healthy and is not likely to bring you lasting happiness. Under these circumstances, put your sobriety first and get off the emotional roller coaster as fast as possible. The tormented feelings these relationships engender have nothing to do with real love. Despite your unreasonable fixation with the person, nothing of value will be lost if you walk away.

A Long-Range Plan

To newly recovering alcoholics, life's daily challenges can be so painful that long-term goals can easily be pushed aside. At the Health Recovery Center, we encourage clients to think ahead and set their sights on goals they may have abandoned years ago. One technique that works more often than you might suspect is keeping a diary of your thoughts. Use it to put your hopes and dreams in writing and converse honestly with yourself about the direction of your life. Over time, you should find that certain themes keep recurring. Your focus on your future will become clearer, and you can begin to plan how to get from here to there. Bear in mind that most long-range goals are met not by big leaps but by small steps that slowly but surely bring you closer and closer to your destination. The secret is mental perseverance. Name your dreams and then hang on to them.

To affirm your plans for the future, use Chart 13 to outline your personal aftercare plan. As you put it into effect, day by day, remember that your goal is improvement, not perfection.

Relapse Insurance

The principal cause of alcoholic relapse can be summed up in one word: cravings. Earlier in this chapter I discussed primary and secondary addictive desires and the factors that can trigger them. In these closing pages I want to reemphasize and summarize them. If you take nothing else away from this book, please bear in mind the triggers that can fire your craving for alcohol.

A *primary* need to drink is an intense, nearly unavoidable involuntary urge. It can be set off by a hypoglycemic drop in glucose, by food or chemical sensitivities, or by poor nutritional habits. Prescription drugs, over-the-counter medications, caffeine, and nicotine can trigger cravings. For comfortable sobriety you must avoid refined sugar, white flour, processed and convenience foods, and, if you are allergic, those foods that elicit reactions. Frequent small meals, rest, and exercise as well as nutritional supplements will provide your body with the

Chart 13. My One-Year Aftercare Plan

1. Physical Goals

Avoiding drugs:

Diet:

Exercise plan:

Maintenance nutrient program:

Medical appointments:

Other:

2. Psychological Goals

Support system choice:

Therapy needs:

New friendships:

Other:

3. Personal Growth

Spiritual needs:

Career choices:

Relationship goals:

Educational needs:

Other:

4. Long-Range Goals

(Sign here) _____

strength to deal with unwanted stress and support the healing process.

Secondary triggers are situations associated with your drinking behavior of the past. Restaurants, parties, and any other settings where you formerly used alcohol can cue you to drink. So can intense negative emotions—anger, self-pity, depression, and fear. The tools of rational-emotive therapy (see Appendix B for suggested books) can help you establish new perceptions and methods of self-direction. The support system you construct—a sponsor, AA, sober friends, recreation, rewarding work—are essential for recovery and will protect and nurture you as you heal physically. Eroding this safe life-style by abandoning the tools you have learned will leave you without protection. It is then only a matter of time before alcoholism reclaims you. If you do stumble down that road someday, remember that you still have, between the covers of this book, a map that will guide you back to safe ground. Sobriety is a lifelong commitment, and it takes time for new habits to become second nature. Your aftercare plan is actually a checklist of relapse-prevention strategies. Review it often and follow it faithfully.

Total Repair:
Treatment Model of the Future

What you have learned from this book represents the early stages of a new and remarkable approach to the treatment of alcoholism. As I write, the search for more biochemical knowledge to help combat this deadly disease is accelerating. Each year, scientists learn more, and each year we make more breakthroughs toward finding the causes and cures for addiction.

I am confident that in the years to come the recovery program described in this book will be the rule rather than the exception in the treatment of alcoholism. Experience has taught me that the HRC plan is the most realistic and dependable recovery strategy available today. I have seen it work for more than ten years. By now, I hope you have come to understand and appreciate the foundation of knowledge upon which it is based. If you have not yet embarked on your treatment plan, I urge you to begin today. You have nothing to lose and everything to gain on your breakthrough journey to health and sobriety. I know you can recover. Now you must discover for yourself how effective this program can be. Godspeed.

A Final Word

In 1987, the nonprofit Rob Mathews Memorial Foundation was established in memory of my son. It has a threefold purpose:

- To study new methods of biochemical repair
- To offer treatment that includes biochemical restoration to impoverished alcoholics
- To educate professionals about our approach and train them to use the techniques effectively

The foundation welcomes any gifts, no matter how small, to continue this work. I like to think that Rob would be proud of the changes in treatment inspired by his short life and tragic death.

Rob Mathews Memorial Foundation
3255 Hennepin Avenue South, Suite 100
Minneapolis, MN 55408
(612)827-7800

Appendix A
References

Foreword

J. S. Goodwin and J. M. Goodwin, "The Tomato Effect: Rejection of Highly Effective Therapies," *Journal of the American Medical Association* 251, (1984):2387–90.

Chapter 2

M. B. Kendell and M. C. Staten, "The Fate of Untreated Alcoholics," *Quarterly Journal of Studies on Alcohol* 27(1966):30–41.

F. LaMere, "What Happens to Alcoholics," *American Journal of Psychiatry* 109(1953):674–76.

K. Powell et al., "Comparison of Three Outpatient Treatment Interventions: A Twelve Month Follow-up of Men Alcoholics," *Quarterly Journal of Studies on Alcohol* 46, no. 4(1985):309–12.

D. Gerard and G. Saenger, "The Abstinent Alcoholic," *Archives of General Psychiatry* 6(1962):83–95.

C. D. Emrich, "A Review of Psychologically Oriented Treatments of Alcoholism, I," *Quarterly Journal of Studies on Alcohol* 35(1974):523–49.

———, "A Review of Psychologically Oriented Treatments of Alcoholism, II," *Quarterly Journal of Studies on Alcohol* 36(1975):88–107.

V. Polich, D. Armor, and H. Braiker, *The Course of Alcoholism, Four Years after Treatment* (Santa Monica, Calif.: Rand Corporation, 1980):169–70.

George Vaillant, *The Natural History of Alcoholism* (Cambridge, Mass.: Harvard University Press, 1983), 285.

Diagnostic and Statistical Manual of Mental Disorders, 3d ed. (Washington, D.C.: American Psychiatric Association, 1980).

"A New Agenda for Alcohol Research: The Institute of Medicine Report on Causes and Consequences," *Alcohol Word* 13, no. 2(1989):183–92.

S. Pell and C. D. Alonzo, "A Five Year Mortality Study of Alcoholics," *Journal of Occupational Medicine* 15(Feb. 1973):120–25.

M. Berglund, "Suicide in Alcoholism," *Archives of General Psychiatry* 41(1984):888–91.

Gerard and Saenger, "The Abstinent Alcoholic," 44–47.

C. DeSoto et al., "Alcoholics at Various Stages of Symptomology in Abstinence," *Alcoholism, Clinical and Experimental Research* 9(Dec. 1985):505–12.

Polich, Armor, and Braiker, *Course of Alcoholism,* 159–70.

E. Gordis, "What is Alcoholism Research?" *Annals of Internal Medicine* 85(1976):821–23.

M. B. Sobell and L. C. Sobell, "Alcoholics Treated by Individualized Behavior Therapy: One Year Treatment Outcome," *Behavior Research and Therapy* 11(1973):599–618.

"Drinking by Alcoholics? New Findings and a Reevaluation of a Major Affirmative Study," *Science* 217(Feb. 1982):169–75.

J. Helzer et al., "The Extent of Long Term Moderate Drinking Among Alcoholics Discharged from Medical and Psychiatric Treatment Facilities," *New England Journal of Medicine* (June 27, 1985):1678–82.

William Mayer, "Differentiating Alcohol Abuse and Alcoholism," *Alcoholism Magazine* (May 1982):51.

U.S. Fourth District Court of Minnesota Decision: Granville House, Inc. Plaintiff vs. Dept. of Health and Human Services, et al., Defendants (Nov. 10, 1982):1–23.

Chapter 3

D. W. Goodwin, "Alcoholism and Heredity," *Archives of General Psychiatry* 36(1979):57–61.

D. W. Goodwin et al., "Alcohol Problems in Adoptees Raised Apart from Biological Parents," *Archives of General Psychiatry* 28, (1973):238–43.

C. R. Cloninger, M. Bohman, and S. Sigvardsson, "Inheritance of Alcohol Abuse: Cross Fostering Analyses of Adopted Men," *Archives of General Psychiatry* 38(1981):861–68.

R. J. Cadoret, C. A. Cain, and W. M. Grove, "Development of Alcoholism in Adoptees Raised Apart from Alcoholic Biologic Relatives," *Archives of General Psychiatry* 37(1980):563.

H. Begleiter, transcript of "Alcoholism: Life Under the Influence," PBS TV *Nova,* No. 1021, January 10, 1984.

L. Tunglai et al., "Isolation of II Alcohol Hydrogenase of the Human Liver: A Determinant of Alcoholism," *Proceedings of the National Academy of Science U.S.A.* 74, no. 10(Oct. 1977):4378–81.

J. A. Ewing, "Studies in the Mechanism of Oriental Hypersensitivity to Alcohol" (Paper presented to the annual meeting of the National Council on Alcoholism, St. Louis, Missouri, September 1978).

"Sobriety in Japan," *Alcoholism Magazine* (May/June 1983):8.

Charles Lieber, "The Metabolism of Alcohol," *Scientific American* 234 (March 1976):31–33.

Marc Schuckit, "Alcoholism and Genetics: Possible Biological Mediators," *Biological Psychiatry* 15, no. 3(1980):437–47.

Virginia Davis and Michael Walsh, "Alcohol, Aminos, Alkaloids: A Possible Biochemical Basis for Alcoholism," *Science* 170 (Dec. 1970):1113–15.

"Born to Drink," *Science Digest* (May 1984):16.

James Tilton and Mark Worden, "The Biogenetics of Alcoholism: Of Mice, Men, and Martinis," *Alcoholism Magazine* (Jan./Feb. 1982):31–33.

Marc Schuckit, "Genetics Possible," *Alcoholism Magazine* (Jan./Feb. 1982).

Theron Randolph and Ralph Moss, *An Alternative Approach to Allergies* (New York: Lippincott & Crowell, 1980), 18–19.

William Philpott and Dwight Kalita, *Brain Allergies: The Psychonutrient Connection* (New Canaan, Conn.: Keats, 1980), 23–24.

Charles Bates, *Depression: The Crucial Role of Nutrition* (Canada: Kask Graphics, 1986), 9–27.

D. Horrobin and M. Manku, "Possible Role of Prostaglandin E_1 in Affective

Disorders and in Alcoholism," *British Medical Journal* (June 1980):1363–66.

D. Horrobin, "Clinical Importance of Essential Fatty Acids" (Paper delivered at the tenth anniversary fall conference of the American College of Advancement in Medicine, Monrovia, Calif., 1983), cassette tape 2, vol. 2.

D. Horrobin, "Prostaglandins (PG_5) and Essential Fatty Acids (EFAs): A New Approach to the Understanding and Treatment of Alcoholism," *Psychiatry in Practice* (Aug. 3, 1984):19–21.

Vaillant, *Natural History of Alcoholism*, 1983.

Vaillant, *Natural History of Alcoholism*, 90–95.

S. Freud, quoted by R. Sackler et al., "Recent Advances in Psychobiology and Their Impact on General Practice," *International Record of Medicine* 170(1957):551.

D. Mossberg et al., "Clinical Conditions in Alcoholics During Long Term Abstinence," *Alcoholism, Clinical and Experimental Research* 8, no. 2(Mar./Apr. 1984):250.

J. Mathews Larson and B. Parker, "Alcoholism Treatment with Biochemical Restoration as a Major Component," *International Journal of Biosocial and Medical Research* 9, no. 1 (1987):92–100.

Chapter 5

P. H. Wolff, "Ethnic Differences in Alcohol Sensitivity," *Science* 175 (1972):449–50.

C. Pfeiffer, *Nutrition and Mental Illness* (Rochester, Vt.: Healing Arts Press, 1975), 40–42.

R. Williams and D. Kalita, *Physician's Handbook on Orthomolecular Medicine* (New York: Pergamon, 1977), 184.

E. Cohen and R. Wurtman, "Brain Acetylcholine: Control by Dietary Choline," *Science* 191(1976):501–62.

Bill Wilson, *A Second Communication to AA Physicians,* 1968. Reprinted by the Huxley Institute for Biosocial Research, 900 North Federal Highway, Boca Raton, FL, 33432.

M. Light, *Hypoglycemia and Me,* 1973. The Hypoglycemia Foundation, 153 Pawling Ave., Troy, NY 12180.

C. Pfeiffer, *Nutrition and Mental Illness,* 18–30.

M. Lesser, *Nutrition and Vitamin Therapy* (New York: Grove Press, 1980), 139–41.

R. Passwater and E. Cranton, *Trace Elements, Hair Analysis, and Nutrition* (New Canaan, Conn.: Keats, 1983).

Chapter 6

F. R. Klenner, "Significance of High Daily Intake of Ascorbic Acid in Preventive Medicine," *Journal of the International Academy of Preventive Medicine* 1 (1974):45–69.

A. Kalokerinos, *Every Second Child* (New Canaan, Conn.: Keats, 1981).

R. F. Cathcart, "Vitamin C: Treating to Bowel Tolerance, Anascorbemia, and Acute Induced Scurvy," *Medical Hypothesis* 7(1974):1359–76.

I. Stone, *The Healing Factor: Vitamin C Against Disease* (New York: Grosset & Dunlap, 1970).

A. Libby and I. Stone, "The Hypoascorbemia-Kwashiorkor Approach to Drug Addiction Therapy: A Pilot Study," *Journal of Orthomolecular Psychiatry* 6, no. 4 (1977):5.

Williams and Kalita, *Orthomolecular Medicine,* 58.

L. Mueller and K. Ketcham, *Eating Right to Live Sober* (Seattle: Madrona, 1983), 253.

"Magnesium Can Help the Alcoholic," *Prevention* (Nov. 1968):73–78.

R. Goodhart, "The Role of Nutritional Factors in the Cause, Prevention and Cure of Alcoholism," *American Journal of Clinical Nutrition* 5(1957):612.

Libby and Stone, "Hypoascorbemia-Kwashiorkor Approach," 5.

L. L. Rogers and R. B. Pelton, "Glutamine in the Treatment of Alcoholism," *Quarterly Journal of Studies on Alcohol* 18, no. 4 (1957):581–87.

E. R. Braverman and C. Pfeiffer, *The Healing Nutrients Within* (New Canaan, Conn.: Keats, 1987), 83.

K. Blum and M. Trachtenberg, "Neurochemistry and Alcohol Craving," *California Society for Treatment of Alcoholism News* 13, no. 2 (September 1986):3.

G. Edwards and J. Littleton, eds., *Pharmacological Treatments for Alcoholism* (London: Croon Heim, 1984), 331–50.

D. J. Segarnick et al., "Biochemical and Behavioral Interactions Between PGE$_1$ and Alcohol," in D. Horrobin, ed., *Clinical Uses of Essential Fatty Acids* (Montreal: Eden Press, 1982), 199–204.

E. Glen et al., "Pharmacological Approaches to the Prevention and Treatment of Alcohol Related CNS Impairment: Results of Double-Blind Trial of Essential Fatty Acids," in Edwards and Littleton, *Pharmacological Treatments for Alcoholism,* 331–50.

D. E. Wilson et al., "Prostaglandin E₁ Prevents Alcohol-Induced Fatty Liver," *Clinical Resources* 21(1973):829.

R. Smith, "A Five-Year Trial of Massive Nicotinic Acid Therapy of Alcoholics in Michigan," *Journal of Orthomolecular Psychiatry* 3(1974):327–31.

M. Schuckit, "Alcohol and Drug Interactions with Anti-Anxiety Medications," *American Journal of Medicine* 82 (May 22, 1987).

Chapter 7

J. Tintera, "Stabilizing Homeostasis in the Recovering Alcoholic Through Endocrine Therapy: Evaluation of the Hypoglycemic Factor," *Journal of American Geriatrics* 14, no. 2(1966):71, 90, 92.

Bill Wilson, *Second Communication to AA Physicians,* 31–33.

Linda Shaw, "Junkie Food," *Prevention* (April 1980):89–91.

J. Poulos, D. Stafford, and K. Carron, *Alcoholism, Stress, and Hypoglycemia* (New York: Sterling, 1976), 95.

M. Worden and G. Rosselini, "The Dry Drunk Syndrome: A Toximolecular Interpretation," *Journal of Orthomolecular Psychiatry* 9, no. 1 (1980):41–44.

E. Cheraskin and W. Ringsdorf, *New Hope for Incurable Diseases* (New York: Arco, 1971), 61–62.

G. Dhopeshwarkar, *Nutrition and Brain Development* (New York: Plenum, 1983), 23.

J. Cohen, "Hypoglycemia and Liver Disease Category II: Fed State Post-Prandial Hypoglycemia with No Evidence of Disturbed Liver Function," *Annals of the New York Academy of Sciences* 273(1976):340.

F. Hale et al., "Post-Prandial Hypoglycemia," *Journal of Biological Psychiatry* 17(1982):125–30.

C. Fredericks, *Psycho-Nutrition* (New York: Grosset & Dunlap, 1976), 128–30.

M. Wellman, "The Late Withdrawal Symptoms of Alcoholic Addiction," *Canadian Medical Association Journal* 70(1954):526–30.

R. J. Solberg, *The Dry Drunk Syndrome* (Center City, Minn.: Hazelden Foundation, 1977).

E. M. Jellinek, "The Withdrawal Syndrome in Alcoholism," *Canadian Medical Association Journal* 81(1959):536–41.

Worden and Rossolini, "The Dry Drunk Syndrome," 44.

Fredericks, *Psycho-Nutrition,* 129–31.

Williams and Kalita, *Orthomolecular Medicine,* 157–58.

J. Tintera, *Hypoadrenocorticism* (Mt. Vernon, N.Y.: Hypoglycemia Foundation, 1974), 71–72.

Wilson, *Second Communication to AA Physicians,* 1–14, 31–32.

Abram Hoffer, *Orthomolecular Medicine for Physicians* (New Canaan, Conn.: Keats, 1989), 37.

Williams and Kalita, *Orthomolecular Medicine,* 185.

Magnesium Bulletin 4, no. 2(1982), as reported in M. R. Werbach, *Nutritional Influences on Illness* (New Canaan, Conn.: Keats, 1988), 242.

A. S. Abraham et al., *American Journal of Clinical Nutrition* 33 (1980):2294–98.

Williams, 184.

Arnold Fox, "Caffeine: Unexpected Causes of Fatigue," *Let's Live* (April 1982):20.

Pfeiffer, *Nutrition and Mental Illness,* 18–32.

Passwater and Cranton, *Trace Elements,* 272–84.

Ibid., 254, 264.

S. Levine and P. Kidd, *Antioxidant Adaptation: Its Role in Free Radical Pathology* (San Leandro, Calif.: Biocurrents Division, Allergy Research Group, 1985), 1–20.

R. Rudin and C. Felix, *The Omega-3 Phenomenon: The Nutritional Breakthrough of the 80's* (New York: Rawson Assoc., 1987).

Chapter 8

C. Lieber et al., "Alcohol Induced Changes in Amino Acid and Protein Metabolism," in *Medical Disorders of Alcoholism: Pathogenesis and Treatment* (Philadelphia: W.B. Saunders, 1982), 178–236.

C. Pfeiffer, *Mental and Elemental Nutrients* (New Canaan, Conn.: Keats, 1975), 158, 163.

Edwards and Littleton, *Pharmacological Treatments for Alcoholism,* 331–50.

H. Salmi and S. Sarna, "Effect of Silymarin on Chemical, Functional, and Morphological Alterations of the Liver: A Double-Blind Study," *Scandinavian Journal of Gastroenterology* 17 (1982):517–21.

L. Benda et al., "The Influence of Therapy with Silymarin on Survival Rate of Patients with Liver Cirrhosis," *Wiener Klinische Wochen-Schrift* (Oct. 10, 1980):678.

Pfeiffer, *Mental and Elemental Nutrients,* 424.

C. Pfeiffer, *The Schizophrenias: Ours to Conquer* (Wichita: Bio Communications Press, 1988), 134–38.

J. Yaryura-Tobias, "L-Tryptophan in Obsessive-Compulsive Disorders," *American Journal of Psychiatry* 10 (Nov. 1977):1298–99.

Passwater and Cranton, *Trace Elements,* 245–88.

A. Keys et al., *The Biology of Human Starvation* (Minneapolis: University of Minnesota Press, 1950).

A. Libby and I. Stone, "The Hyperascorbemia-Kwashiorkor Approach to Drug Addiction: A Pilot Study," *Journal of Orthomolecular Medicine* 6, no. 4(1977).

Braverman and Pfeiffer, *Healing Nutrients Within,* 23.

Ibid., 197.

R. Erdman, *The Amino Revolution* (Chicago: Contemporary Books, 1987), 33.

Ibid., 92–93.

W. Repogle and F. Eicke, "Megavitamin Therapy in the Reduction of Anxiety and Depression Among Alcoholics," *Journal of Orthomolecular Medicine* 4, no. 4(1989):221–24.

Lesser, *Nutrition and Vitamin Therapy,* 69–70.

Erdman, *Amino Revolution,* 100.

Lesser, *Nutrition and Vitamin Therapy,* 69–70.

M. Werbach, *Nutritional Influences on Illness,* 17–18.

"Researcher Links Depression to Deficiency of Two Chemicals," *Minneapolis Star Tribune,* Oct. 29, 1983, section 1B, p. 1, col. 1–2.

Cohen and Wurtman, "Brain Acetylcholine," 501–62.

Pfeiffer, *Mental and Elemental Nutrients,* 173–77.

Dhopeshwarkar, *Nutrition and Brain Development,* 89.

H.L. Newbold, *Meganutrients for Your Nerves* (New York: Wyden, 1975), 344.

E. Colby-Morley, "Neurotransmitters and Nutrition," *Journal of Orthomolecular Psychiatry* 12, no.1(1983):39.

Pfeiffer, *Mental and Elemental Nutrients,* 138–51.

Mueller and Ketcham, *Eating Right to Live Sober,* 256.

Tintera, *Hypoadrenocorticism,* 130–34.

Tintera, "Stabilizing Homeostasis," 71–96.

Erdman, *Amino Revolution,* 24, 37.

Philpott and Kalita, *Brain Allergies,* 66.

Lesser, *Nutrition and Vitamin Therapy,* 48–95.

Braverman and Pfeiffer, *Healing Nutrients Within,* 39.

K. Budd, "Use of D-Phenylalanine, An Enkephalinase Inhibitor, in the Treatment of Intractable Pain," *Advanced Pain Research Therapy* (1983):305–8.

J. Bonica et al., eds. *Advances in Pain Research and Therapy,* vol. 5 (New York: Raven Press, 1983), 289–93.

Braverman and Pfeiffer, *Healing Nutrients Within,* 42, 67.

Ibid., 132.

Goodhart, "Nutritional Factors in the Cause, Prevention, and Cure of Alcoholism," 612.

Mueller and Ketcham, *Eating Right to Live Sober,* 71–72.

Glenn et al., "Prevention and Treatment of Alcohol-related CNS Impairment," 331–50.

Chapter 9

A. Hoffer, "Mechanism of Action of Nicotinic Acid in the Treatment of Schizophrenia," in D. Hawkins and L. Pauling, eds., *Orthomolecular Psychiatry* (San Francisco: Freeman and Co., 1973), 239.

R. Bolton, "Aggression and Hypoglycemia Among the Quolla: A Study in Psychobiological Anthropology," *Ethnology* 12(July 1973):227.

W. Herbert, "The Case of the Missing Hormones," *Science News* (October 30, 1982):282.

Braverman and Pfeiffer, *Healing Nutrients Within,* 120–36.

D. Pearson and S. Shaw, *The Life Extension Companion* (New York: Warner Books, 1983).

Pfeiffer, *Nutrition and Mental Illness,* 26–32.

A. Schauss, *Diet, Crime and Delinquency* (Berkeley: Parker House, 1980).

Erdman, The *Amino Revolution,* 105–6.

Horrobin, "Clinical Importance of Essential Fatty Acids," tape 2.

Hoffer, *Orthomolecular Medicine,* 160–62.

M. Victor, R. Adams, and G. Collins, *The Wernicke-Korsakoff Syndrome* (Philadelphia: F. A. Davis, 1971).

D. Pearson, *Life Extension* (New York: Warner Books, 1982), 272.

D. Roe, *Drug Induced Nutritional Deficiencies* (Westport, Conn.: AVI, 1976), 202–6.

H. Tao and H. Fox, "Measurement of Urinary Pantothenic Acid Excretion of Alcoholic Patients," *Journal of Nutritional Science* 22(1976):333–37.

Chapter 10

Colby-Morley, "Neurotransmitters and Nutrition," 38–43.

M.J.A.J.M. Hoes, "L-Tryptophan in Depression," *Journal of Orthomolecular Psychiatry* 4(1982):231.

A. Coppen et al., *Archives of General Psychiatry* 26(1972):234.

J. Fernstrom and R. Wurtman, "Brain Serotonin Content: Physiological Dependence on Plasma Tryptophan Levels," *Science* 173(1971):149–52.

A. Gelenberg et al., "Tyrosine for the Treatment of Depression," *American Journal of Psychiatry* 137, no. 5(1980):622–23.

I. Goldberg, "Tyrosine in Depression," *Lancet* 2(1980):364.

H. Beckman et al., "DL-Phenylalanine Versus Imipramine: A Double-blind Controlled Study," *Archiv fur Psychiatre und Nerven Krankheiten* 227(1979):49–58.

H. Beckman, "Phenylalanine in Affective Disorders," *Advanced Biological Psychiatry* 10(1983):137–47.

C. Bates, *Essential Fatty Acids, Immunity and Mental Health* (Tacoma, Wa.: Life Sciences Press).

Werbach, *Nutritional Influences on Illness,* 159–60.

D. Horrobin and M. Manku, "Prostaglandin E_1 in Affective Disorders and in Alcoholism," 1363–66.

Newbold, *Meganutrients for Your Nerves,* 19.

M. Carney et al., "Thiamine, Riboflavin and Pyridoxine Deficiency in Psychiatric Inpatients," *British Journal of Psychiatry* 141(1982):271–72.

E. Lieber, "Alcohol and Nutrition," *Alcohol World* 13, no. 3(1989).

D. Zucker et al., "B_{12} Deficiency and Psychiatric Disorders," *Biologic Psychiatry* 16(1981):197–205.

Werbach, *Nutritional Influences on Illness,* 155–158.

Passwater and Cranton, *Trace Elements,* 31, 64, 105, 122, 161.

W. Webb and M. Gehe, "Electrolyte and Fluid Imbalance: Neuropsychiatric Manifestations," *Psychosomatics* 3(1981):199–203.

B. Barnes, *Hypothyroidism: The Unsuspected Illness* (New York: Harper & Row, 1976).

J. Rippon, *Medical Mycology,* 2d ed. (Philadelphia: W.B. Saunders, 1982).

H. Van Praag, "Depression, Suicide and the Metabolism of Serotonin in the Brain," *Journal of Affective Disorders* 4(1982):275–90.

Chapter 11

Randolph and Moss, *Alternative Approach to Allergies,* 30.

P. Saifer and M. Zellerbach, *Detox* (New York: St. Martin's Press, 1984).

Philpott and Kalita, *Brain Allergies,* 23–25.

A. Schauss and C. Costin, *Zinc and Eating Disorders* (New Canaan, Conn.: Keats, 1989), 22–28.

A. S. Prasad, "Zinc Deficiency in Man," *American Journal of Disturbed Children* 130(1976):259–61.

D. Bhattacharyas et al., "Significantly Altered Copper and Zinc Levels in Serum, Urine, Liver, and Skeletal Muscle of Morbidly Obese Patients," *Journal of the American College of Nutrition* 7(1988):401.

K. Sehnert, *The Garden Within* (Burlingame, Calif.: Health World, Inc., 1989), 39.

G. Kroker, "Chronic Candidiasis and Allergy," in J. Brostoff and S. Callencorte, eds., *Food Allergy and Intolerance* (London: Bailliere Tindahl, 1987), 850–72.

K. Iwata, "A Review of the Literature on Drunken Symptoms Due to Yeasts in the Gastrointestinal Tract," *Yeast and Yeast-Like Microorganisms in Medical Science* (Tokyo: University of Tokyo Press, 1972), 260–68.

W. Crook, *The Yeast Connection,* 3d ed. (Jackson, Tenn.: Professional Books, 1983), 30–33.

J. Trowbridge and M. Walker, *The Yeast Syndrome* (New York: Bantam Books, 1986), 69.

K. Sehnert and J. Mathews Larson, "Candida-Related Complex (CRC), a Complicating Factor in Treatment and Diagnostic Screening for Alcoholics: A Pilot Study of 213 Patients," *International Journal of Biosocial and Medical Research* 13(1991):67–76.

Chapter 12

Journal of Addictive Behavior 3(1978):13–15.

"Problem Drinkers are Smokers," *Journal of Studies on Alcohol* 37(Sept. 1976):1316.

Braverman, *Healing Nutrients Within,* 191–210.

Appendix B
Suggested Reading

Alcoholism (Biological Orientation)

How to Defeat Alcoholism, by Joseph Beasley (New York: Times Books, 1989).

Under the Influence, by James Milam (Seattle: Madrona Press, 1981).

Eating Right to Live Sober, by Ann Mueller and Katherine Ketcham (Seattle: Madrona Press, 1983).

The Prevention of Alcoholism Through Nutrition, by Roger J. Williams (New York: Bantam, 1981).

Wrong Diagnosis, Wrong Treatment, by Joseph Beasley (New York: Creative Informatics, 1987).

The Hidden Addiction, by Janice Phelps (Boston: Little, Brown & Co., 1986).

A Second Communication to AA Physicians, by Bill Wilson. The 1968 reprint can be purchased from the Huxley Institute for Biosocial Research, 900 North Federal Highway, Boca Raton, FL 33432.

Hypoglycemia

Low Blood Sugar and You, by Carlton Fredricks (New York: Constellation International, 1969).

Pure, White, and Deadly, by John Yudkin (New York: Viking, 1986).

The Sugar Trap and How to Avoid It, by Beatrice Trum-Hunter (Boston: Houghton-Mifflin, 1982).

Sugar Blues, by William Dufty (New York: Warner, 1976).

Hypoglycemia: The Disease Your Doctor Won't Treat, by Harvey Ross and Jeraldine Saunders (New York: Pinnacle Books, 1989).

Allergies

Allergies and Your Family, by Doris Rapp (New York: Sterling Publishing Co., 1981).

An Alternative Approach to Allergies, by Theron Randolph and Ralph Moss (New York: Lippincott & Crowell, 1980).

Brain Allergies: The Psychonutrient Connection, by William Philpott and Dwight Kalita (New Canaan, Conn.: Keats, 1980).

Detox, by Phyllis Saifer (Los Angeles: Tarcher, 1984).

The Type 1/Type 2 Allergy Relief Program, by Alan Levin (Los Angeles: Tarcher, 1983).

Human Ecology and Susceptibility to the Chemical Environment, by Theron Randolph (Springfield, Ill.: Charles Thomas, 1962).

Coping with Your Allergies, by Natalie Golos (New York: Simon & Schuster, 1979).

Chemical Additives in Booze, by Michael Lipske (Washington, D.C.: Center for Science in the Public Interest, 1982).

Nutrition

Feed Yourself Right, by Lendon Smith (New York: McGraw-Hill, 1983).

Nutrition and Brain Development, by Govind Dhopeshwarkar, (New York: Plenum, 1983).

Diet for a Small Planet, by Frances Moore Lappe (New York: Ballantine, 1971).

Nutrition and Vitamin Therapy, by Michael Lesser (New York: Grove Press, 1980).

Mental and Elemental Nutrients, by Carl Pfeiffer (New Canaan, Conn.: Keats, 1975).

Psychodietetics, by Emanuel Cheraskin (New York: Ringdorf-Bantam, 1976).

Nutrition Against Disease, by Roger Williams (New York: Pitman, 1971).

Medical Applications of Clinical Nutrition, by Jeffrey Bland (New Canaan, Conn.: Keats, 1983).

Great Nutrition Robbery, by Beatrice Trum-Hunter (New York: Scribner's, 1976).

Meganutrients for Your Nerves, by H. L. Newbold (New York: Wyden, 1975).

Depression

The Way Up from Down, by Priscilla Slagle (New York: Random House, 1987).

Health and Light, by John Ott (New York: Simon & Schuster, 1973).

Overcoming Depression, by Paul Hauck (Philadelphia: Westminster Press, 1973).

Candida

The Yeast Connection, by William Crook (Jackson, Tenn.: Professional Books, 1983).

The Yeast Syndrome, by John Trowbridge and Morton Walker (New York: Bantam Books, 1986).

The Missing Diagnosis, by Orien Truss (self-published, 1983). Obtain from P.O. Box 26508, Birmingham, AL 35226.

Rational-Emotive Therapy

A New Guide to Rational Living, by Albert Ellis and Robert Harper (North Hollywood, Calif.:Wilshire Book Co., 1977).

Overcoming Worry and Fear, by Paul Hauck (Philadelphia: Westminster Press, 1975).

Overcoming Jealousy and Possessiveness, by Paul Hauck (Philadelphia: Westminster Press, 1981).

The Self-Talk Solution, by Shad Helmstetter (New York: Pocket Books, 1987).

Psycho-Cybernetics, by Maxwell Maltz (New York: Simon & Schuster, 1966).

Mind as Healer—Mind as Slayer, by Kenneth Pelletier (New York: Dell Publishing, 1977).

Reality Therapy, by William Glasser (New York: Harper & Row, 1965).

Spirituality

The Twelve Steps for Everyone, by Grateful Members (Minneapolis: Compcare Publications, 1975).

Stepping Stones to Recovery, by Bill Pittman (Seattle: Glen Abbey, 1988).

The Promise of a New Day, by Karen Casey and Martha Vanceburg (Center City, Minn.: Hazelden Foundation, 1983).

Man's Search for Meaning, by Victor Frankel (New York: Pocket Books, 1973).

You Can Heal Your Life, by Louise Hay (Santa Monica, Calif.: Hay House, 1984).

Why Am I Afraid to Love?, by John Powell (Niles, Ill.: Argus, 1969).

Appendix C
Recommended Laboratories,
Nutrient Distributors,
and Manufacturers of Nutrients

Laboratories

Company	Tests Performed
Advanced Medicine Nutrition, Inc. 2247 National Avenue Hayward, CA 94540-5012 (800) 437-8888	Hair-analysis lab
Doctor's Data, Inc. P.O. Box 111 30 West 101 Roosevelt Road West Chicago, IL 60185 (312) 231-3649	Hair-analysis lab

Laboratories *(Continued)*

Company	Tests Performed
ImmunoDiagnostic Laboratories P.O. Box 5755 San Leandro, CA 94577 (800) 888-1113 (415) 635-4555	Candida-antibody assays FAMA
Immuno Nutritional Clinical Laboratories 7404 Fulton Avenue, Suite 5 North Hollywood, CA 91605-4114 (800) 344-4646 (818) 780-4720 (in California)	Food-allergy assays Candida-antibody assays
Omegatech P.O. Box 1 Troutdale, VA 24378 (800) 437-1404	Hair-analysis lab
Serammune Physicians' Lab Ltd. 1830 Preston White Drive AMSA Building Reston, VA 22091 (800) 593-5472	Food-allergy assays Candida-antibody assays
Tyson and Associates 12832 Chadron Avenue Hawthorne, CA 90250 (800) 367-7744 (800) 433-9750 (in California)	Amino-acid assays

Nutrient Distributors

Company	Product
Bio Recovery Inc. 3255 Hennepin Avenue South Minneapolis, MN 55408 1-800-24-SOBER	

Manufacturers

Company	Product
Advanced Medical Nutrition, Inc. 2247 National Avenue P.O. Box 5012 Hayward, CA 94540-5012 (415) 783-6969	DL-Phenylalanine
Bio-Therapeutics/Phyto-Pharmacia 510 Lombardi Avenue Green Bay, WI 54305 (800) 553-2370 (414) 435-4200	Nicoril
Cardiovascular Research Ltd./Ecological Formulas 1061-B Shary Circle Concord, CA 94518 (800) 888-4585 (510) 827-3322 (510) 827-2636	Vitamin C (tapioca) Free Radical Quenchers GTF chromium
Ecological Formulas 1061-B Shary Circle Concord, CA 94518 (800) 888-4585 (510) 827-3322 (510) 827-2636	Free Radical Quenchers Ascorbate capsules
Ethical Nutrients of Illinois 20370 North Rand Road Palatine, IL 60074 (800) 523-5294 (708) 438-9420	Cal/Mag Zinc picolinate Chromium picolinate
Murdock Pharmaceuticals 1400 Mountain Springs Parkway Springville, UT 84663 (800) 962-8873	Efamol

Manufacturers *(Continued)*

Company	Product
Natrol, Inc. 26731 Marilla Street Chatsworth, CA 91311 (800) 627-6128 (818) 701-9966	Calm Kids
Nutricology, Inc./Allergy Research Group P.O. Box 489 400 Preda Street San Leandro, CA 94577-0489 (800) 545-9960 (510) 639-4572	Vitamin C (sago palm) Multi Vit/Min Aller-Digest (pancreatic enzymes)
Omega-Life, Inc. 15355 Woodbridge Road Brookfield, WI 53005 (414) 786-2070	Flax
Ominopathy Products 414 North State College Boulevard Anaheim, CA 92806 (800) 627-6128 (714) 538-1540	ACE drops
Richlife-SPI Nutrition 222 N. Vincent Avenue Covina, CA 91722 (800) 533-1038	Niacin (time-release) Lipo-3 Factors (for liver repair)
Twin Laboratories, Inc. 2120 Smithtown Avenue Ronkonkoma, NY 11779 (800) 645-5626	PC-55 (phosphatidylcholine) GABA Plus Glutamine Calcium/magnesium Silymarin

Manufacturers *(Continued)*

Company	Product
Tyson and Associates, Inc. 12832 Chadron Avenue Hawthorne, CA 90250 (800) 367-7744 (800) 433-9750 (in California)	All amino acids

Index

Numerals in *italics* indicate
figures, graphs, and tables.

About the Authors

Joan Mathews Larson, who holds a doctorate in nutrition, is founder of the highly esteemed Health Recovery Center in Minneapolis.

Keith W. Sehnert, M.D., is a respected researcher, former university professor, and well-known medical writer. Medical consultant for the Health Recovery Center, he lives in Minneapolis.